Can You Hear the Clapping of One Hand?

Can You Hear the Clapping of One Hand?

Learning to Live with a Stroke

ILZA VEITH

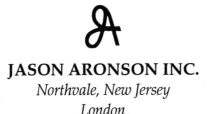

JASON ARONSON INC.
Northvale, New Jersey
London

THE MASTER WORK SERIES

First softcover edition 1997

Copyright © 1997, 1988 by Ilza Veith

All rights reserved. No part of this book may be used or reproduced in any manner whatsoever without written permission from Jason Aronson Inc. except in the case of brief quotations in reviews for inclusion in a magazine, newspaper, or broadcast.

Library of Congress Cataloging-in-Publication Data

Veith, Ilza
    Can you hear the clapping of one hand? : learning to live with a stroke / Ilza Veith
        p. cm. -- (The Master work series)
    Originally published : Berkeley : University of California Press, 1988.
    Includes bibliographical references.
    ISBN 0-7657-0059-X (alk. paper)
    1. Veith, Ilza--Health. 2. Cerebrovascular disease—Patients—United States—Biography. I. Title. II. Series.
    [DNLM: 1. Veith, Ilza. 2. Cerebrovascular Disorders—personal narratives. WL 355 V431c 1997]
RC388.5.V44 1997
362.1'9681—dc21
[B]
DNLM/DLC
for Library of Congress   96-39914

Printed in the United States of America on acid-free paper. For information and catalog write to Jason Aronson Inc., 230 Livingston Street, Northvale, New Jersey 07647-1731. Or visit our website: http://www.aronson.com

In memory of Hans
A Man for All Seasons

Contents

	Foreword	ix
	Preface to the Softcover Edition	xiii
	Preface	xv
	Acknowledgments	xvii
1.	Perspective	1
2.	My Single Hand and Early Tears	4
	The Cerebral Vascular Accident 10	
3.	The Event: Functions Lost and Retained	13
4.	The Hospital: Tender, Loving Care?	20
	Brain Scan and the Mirage of Recovery 28	
	The Horror of the Carotid Angiogram 30	
	Physical Therapy: To Stand on Both Feet 36	
	Hospital Visitors, Flowers, and Futile Comfort 41	
	Gadgets for Recovery 43	
5.	Return Home	48
	Routine of Daily Life 51	

　　　　Resumption of Work at the
　　　　　University　52
　　　　Convalescence Open-Ended　58
　　　　Recovery by Surgery　60
　　　　The Specter of Overweight　63
　　　　Learning to Cope　66
　　　　Pain and Acupuncture Therapy　71

6.　Dreams: Hopeful and Threatening　　　　　78

7.　Afterthoughts　　　　　　　　　　　　　　87

　　Glossary　　　　　　　　　　　　　　　　97

Foreword

Ilza Veith had only recently joined the faculty of a major university and had become a noted historian of health sciences and psychiatry. Years of productivity lay ahead for her. A stroke, which paralyzed the left side of her body, clouded Dr. Veith's bright future. It also altered her view of life and people. Today, twenty years later, she is still enraged over the blow that life dealt her.

Can You Hear the Clapping of One Hand? is the author's creative way of coping with anger that will not go away. "This book . . . is written from an inner need, with the hope that by writing about my stroke and all the grief and pain it has caused me, I may be able to abreact some of my anger and resentment," Dr. Veith writes.

It is with this book that Ilza Veith does what we in psychiatry call her "grief work," learning to cope with the loss of a loved one. Ilza Veith lost a part of herself. Her book is filled with anger; her descriptions of maltreating her visitors until some stopped coming can be of benefit to the reader intent on a clinical examination of the dynamics of strokes.

This is not ordinary grief work but is in keeping with Dr. Veith's persona; it is grief work with a purpose and a product. For teaching the public about this illness and its victims has become a major focus of Ilza Veith's life, first in lectures before university departments of the neurosciences, and now, with the writing of this book. It is a work that can be a learning experience for health professionals and laymen alike.

Let me express my reactions to the book by noting those with whom I shared them and my reasons for doing so:

> Neurologists—to assess possible new insights that Ilza Veith's disciplined and excellent description of symptoms may elicit.
>
> Patients—to gauge how they might learn skills that would be helpful and to learn new ways of managing the physical and mental part of the disease.
>
> Psychiatrists—to become knowledgeable about the complex nature of emotional and cognitive reactions to functional loss through a stroke.
>
> Social workers—to note the key roles of spouses and families.
>
> Rehabilitation specialists, surgeons, and others—to encourage them to use their skills to the maximum.
>
> My daughter, Laurie, a physician in physical medicine rehabilitation—to further her education as no other book I know can do.

This book will be of interest to anyone concerned with the human condition. One of its strengths is the author's painful reminder of what it is like to be a patient, helpless in the face of strangers and instruments that poke at and prick you. There are lessons here for visitors, whose efforts at cheering up a grieving patient can be grating and may elicit angry responses. Pain and grief must be acknowledged. You could never tell Ilza Veith that, in any case, she still had her right arm—and get away with it.

Foreword

The victim-author has much to say about patients' dependence and independence and the efficacy of various therapies, including the one that attempts to teach the handicapped to be independent by refusing to help them even in accord with what normal courtesy would require.

But perhaps, above all, this book is a story of hope. "Strangely . . . I responded to the challenge of helplessness by being even more productive than in my previous healthy years," Veith writes. "I was simply incapable of giving up all hope."

I am glad Ilza Veith never gave up hope, for her sake and for all our sakes.

Bertram S. Brown, M.D.

President and Chief Executive Officer
Hahnemann University
Philadelphia, Pa.

Preface to the Softcover Edition

This is a personal book. I am a medical doctor but I am also a patient, the victim of a severe hemiplegia that has left the left side of my body immobile. A gratifying result of the first edition of this book about my own stroke was the letters from readers who responded to this little book in a very personal way. Some were from people who had suffered a stroke themselves. Others were from those who loved and cared for them. Thirty-four years have now passed since I suffered my stroke. I still walk with a limp, feel severe pain on my left side from the ankle to the knee, and from there into the hip. It is a great happiness to me that my account of my own experiences with a massive stroke may have helped give readers the strength to soldier on, as I also have done.

Everyone needs support. The first edition of this book was dedicated to my husband Hans, whose tireless support and extraordinary devotion helped me cope with the deprivation, discomfort, and handicaps resulting from the hemiplegia. Now I dedicate this new edition to Hans's memory. He died at home of a slow and painful ailment, at the age of ninety-two. Because of my impairment there was little I could do personally to nurse him or alleviate his suffering. I could and did pass hours at his bedside trying to distract him and cheer him up. For nursing care at home we depended on a young cheerful Chinese woman with whom we both immediately established friendly contact. Lucy also grew accustomed to helping me during my husband's illness and now remains with me full-time for as long as necessary.

In other respects I have not been so fortunate. Like some of my readers I have felt the rejection that a stroke can bring about. For years I was vice-chairman of the Department of the History of Health Sciences at the University of California Medical School in San Francisco. My chairman remained satisfied with my performance in this position after my stroke. Even after retirement I retained the use of an office at the university. All this changed with the retirement of my chairman and the arrival of his successor. Though he had known me for some years he sent me an official notice that I must vacate my office immediately because it was needed for newly arriving faculty. If I did not do so immediately he would have professional movers move everything, including my publications and years of professional correspondence, at my expense. In my haste to obviate this threat a good many items were lost or mislaid.

In spite of this irreplaceable loss, but thanks to my own extensive professional library, I have found it possible to continue my scholarly publications; I travel widely and continue to give lectures at home and abroad. I too soldier on as well as I can. I wish my reader well.

Preface

This book was written in the hope that it will be of interest and use to neuroscientists, to other stroke victims, and to all those whose families include a hemiplegic member. Like several other stroke victims,* I felt the urge to write about my illness since it happened in 1964 and left me paralyzed on my left side. In the intervening twenty-four years I have come to realize that stroke, although far from being a rare and exotic affliction, is essentially not very well known in all its variations by the medical profession, still less known by sufferers from that illness, and even less by the general public, which tends to assume that all strokes are alike and that almost any excited person with a temporarily florid complexion looks as though he or she were on the verge of apoplexy.

Very few people, including neurologists and general physicians, have an intimate knowledge of the event of suffering a stroke and the arduous process of physical and emotional recovery; but most people—middle-aged or elderly—when confronted with a stroke victim seem

---

*Agnes De Mille, *Reprieve, A Memoir*. Garden City, New York: Doubleday & Company, 1981; Eric Hodgins, *Episode, Report on the Accident Inside My Skull*. New York: Atheneum, 1964.

apprehensive that they too might be potential victims of that fearsome affliction and are usually very much interested in hearing my story. In fact, several university departments of the neurosciences even invited me to speak about "my" stroke to members of their faculty, their residents, interns, senior students, and even to some of their patients who were sufficiently recovered to attend an hour's instructive discourse. From the lively discussions that usually followed my lectures, I could gauge the avid interest of the audience in my melancholy subject.

Although I did not keep a diary of my illness, the diagnostic investigations, and the attempts at recovery, I do remember every detail of it so clearly that I found myself able to lecture about my stroke with only a few pages of notes. In writing this book I have followed these lecture notes and my sometimes embarrassing ability of near-total recall that has extended to the various phases of this, the most frightful event in my life. I was encouraged in this undertaking by Bertram S. Brown, M.D., the former director of the National Institute of Mental Health, and currently president and chief executive officer of Hahnemann University in Philadelphia. At the time Dr. Brown urged me to carry out my intention to write all this down, his interest and compassion in physical disability were heightened because of his experiences as a member of the U.S. Council for Disabled Persons.

Acknowledgments

While I alone conceived the idea of making my illness the subject of this book, I could not have done it without the support of several people who have made my life possible, and at times even enjoyable, during the two decades of my hemiplegia. Strangely, it was during these years that I responded to the challenge of my helplessness by being more productive than in many previously healthy years.

Above all, I wish to record my endless gratitude to my husband, Hans, to whom this book is dedicated. He is truly "a man for all seasons." He has lent me not only a hand, but often both hands, while I had the use of only one.

I further wish to thank my colleagues and chiefs at the University of California, San Francisco. Chancellor Emeritus J. B. de C. M. Saunders, M.D., upon whose invitation I had joined the faculty of the university. During the early period of my illness and hospitalization he did not let a day go by without paying me a visit in my hospital room. I thank both him and Professor Gert H. Brieger for having shown great consideration for the restrictions imposed upon me by my handicap.

Similar forbearance was shown me by all my students who became, and have remained, my friends. I wish to thank them for their affection and patience with their handicapped teacher.

Finally, I express my gratitude to my dear friend Francis Schiller, M.D., a gifted colleague in the history of health sciences and a compassionate neurologist who gave me his time to criticize and discuss almost every sentence of this book.

Notes on Names

Although this book is a factual account of my illness, I have altered and fictionalized all the names, except for those in the anecdote about Anna Freud and the names used in the Acknowledgments.

San Francisco Ilza Veith
Autumn 1983

Epigraph

The master of Kennin temple was Mokurai, Silent Thunder. He had a little protégé named Toyo who was only twelve years old. Toyo saw the older disciples visit the master's room each morning and evening to receive instruction in sanzen or personal guidance in which they were given koans to stop mind-wandering.

Toyo wished to do sanzen also.

"Wait a while," said Mokurai. "You are too young."

But the child insisted, so the teacher finally consented.

In the evening little Toyo went at the proper time to the threshold of Mokurai's sanzen room. He struck the gong to announce his presence, bowed respectfully three times outside the door, and went to sit before the master in respectful silence.

"You can hear the sound of two hands when they clap together," said Mokurai. "Now show me the sound of one hand."

Toyo bowed and went to his room to consider this problem. From his window he could hear the music of the geishas. "Ah, I have it!" he proclaimed.

The next evening, when his teacher asked him to illustrate the sound of one hand, Toyo began to play the music of the geishas.

"No, no," said Mokurai. "That will never do. That is not the sound of one hand. You've not got it at all."

Thinking that such music might interrupt, Toyo moved his abode to a quiet place. He meditated again. "What can the sound of one hand be?" He happened to hear some water dripping. "I have it," imagined Toyo.

When he next appeared before his teacher, Toyo imitated dripping water.

"What is that?" asked Mokurai. "That is the sound of dripping water, but not the sound of one hand. Try again."

In vain Toyo meditated to hear the sound of one hand. He heard the sighing of the wind. But the sound was rejected.

He heard the cry of an owl. This also was refused.

The sound of one hand was not the locusts.

For more than ten times Toyo visited Mokurai with different sounds. All were wrong. For almost a year he pondered what the sound of one hand might be.

At last little Toyo entered true meditation and transcended all sounds. "I could collect no more," he explained later, "so I reached the soundless sound."

Toyo had realized the sound of one hand.*

Zen Flesh, Zen Bones. A Collection of Zen and Pre-Zen Writings. Compiled by Paul Reps. Charles E. Tuttle Co. Rutland, Vermont, 1957–1968, p. 41.

1
Perspective

At a ceremonious moment during the *Hearings of the U.S. Senate Select Committee on Presidential Campaign Activities,* Senator Sam Ervin interrupted his oratory and decided to place his committee members under renewed oath. "Raise your right hand," he roared proudly along the line of senators. Suddenly he realized that there was one arm lacking among all those raised on this solemn occasion. "Senator Inouye," Ervin said in a ringing voice, "won't you be joining us in raising your right arm?" To the chagrin and acute embarrassment of all participants and the audience, Senator Inouye found himself forced to remain immobile and silent.

It is possible that at this moment Senator Ervin had forgotten what most of those present at the hearing and in the television audience remembered: Senator Inouye had lost his right arm during World War II while serving in the so-called 100th Regiment, and the 442nd Regimental Combat Team that consisted exclusively of Japanese-American volunteer soldiers under General Mark Clark, the Allied commander for the spring campaign in Italy in 1945. These Japanese-American soldiers received 52 Distinguished Service Crosses, 528 Silver Stars, numerous Bronze Stars, Purple Hearts, and other decorations. According to the *Congressional Record* it was the most decorated unit of its size and length of service in the history of the United States. Senator Inouye, unable to raise his right arm on Senator Ervin's command, had received a Distinguished Service Cross, a Bronze Star, and a Purple Heart with Clusters for outstanding bravery and courage.

Evidently, the embarrassing contretemps had left a delayed impression on the chairman and vice chairman of the committee, for on Thursday, August 2, 1973, the official transcript of the meeting of the *U.S. Senate Select Committee on Presidential Campaign Activities* (Book 8, pp. 3,231–3,232) refers to the incident.

After calling the committee to order Senator Ervin spoke as follows:

I am constrained to make some remarks concerning a member of this committee, Senator Danny Inouye of Hawaii. Senator Inouye is an American, a native-born American of Japanese ancestry. I do not know a finer American. He showed his devotion to our country by fighting under its flag, not only for the liberty of our country, but for the liberty of the free world in the Second World War. He suffered severe wounds which necessitated the amputation of his right arm. He was decorated with the Distinguished Service Cross for extraordinary heroism in action with an armed enemy of the United States. And he has proved himself in the latter days as one of the most dedicated Americans this country has ever known, and I feel that events of yesterday make it appropriate for me to make these remarks concerning a member of this committee who has proved himself one of the most gallant of all Americans in the history of this Republic.

When Senator Ervin had concluded his statement, Senator Baker, the committee vice chairman, requested permission to speak on the same subject (pp. 3,231–3,232):

Mr. Chairman, may I say that I have known Danny Inouye since I have been in the Senate. There is no man who is more loyal or dedicated to his country. I do not know anyone on this committee who has made a greater contribution to its efforts than Senator Inouye. I have a great affection for him as well as a great admiration for him. We are in a tension-filled atmosphere and it is unfortunate that things of this sort occur.

I think a mark of Senator Inouye's greatness is that I am sure it will not affect his further consideration of matters that are brought to our attention, and I am sorry that the events of the last several days have occurred. I hope and think that it will not affect the objectivity and the efficiency, the effectiveness, of this committee, and I commend you, Mr. Chairman, for bringing that matter to the attention of the official record, I believe now that it is behind us and we can get on with the business at hand.

The solemn declarations in favor of Senator Inouye concluded that subject for the committee's morning session of August 2, with the exception that Senator Inouye, evidently very moved by the testimonies of his Senate colleagues, asked for permission to address the committee:

Mr. Chairman and Mr. Vice-Chairman, before proceeding I would like to thank both of you for your very generous remarks this morning and, if I may, I would like to take the liberty of thanking you in Hawaiian, *mahalo* and *aloha*, which means thank you very much and I love you both.

2
My Single Hand and Early Tears

I might not have been so much more affected than most television viewers of those Senate hearings probably were had I not also been afflicted with the permanent inability to use one of my hands. Senator Inouye's and my own impairments have always reminded me of one of the best-known Zen enigmas, or koans, by which a Zen master tests the imagination of the Zen disciples. Having spent much time studying in Japan shortly before the awkward contretemps between Ervin and Inouye, I frequently had been exposed to Zen thinking and to the meditation of seemingly insolvable Zen koans. There was one koan which had so far eluded my satori, or comprehension; and now, after the interlude in the Senate hearings, I suddenly understood it: It was the question, "Can you hear the clapping of a single hand?" Now I knew that if public attention had not been directed to it, most viewers would not have noticed the lack of one raised hand.

I was also reminded of the first chamber-music concert I attended after I had lost the use of my left arm and hand. The concert took place in the music room of a large and elegant private home in Chicago, just nine months after I became paralyzed. I was welcomed by all my friends as I slowly made my way into the music room and was told that I looked remarkably well. (Remarkable for what, I thought!) The well-meaning hosts, assuming they were doing me a special favor, had saved a seat for me in the first row of their improvised auditorium, directly in front of the music stands of the cellist and the violinist, both of whom were prominent members of the local symphony orchestra. The major presentation, a concerto for violin and violoncello by Antonio Vivaldi, was played as beautifully as I had remembered their art. At the end of this piece the audience of about one hundred people applauded enthusiastically. In the seat next to me, a woman friend of long standing looked reproachfully at my inactive hands and said in a none-too-soft stage whisper, "Don't you think you should also applaud?" I was somewhat shocked but nodded in her direction and began waving my one usable hand in the rhythm of the applause. The cellist and violinist, both of whom knew me and my impediment, looked at my one waving hand; smiling radiantly and with a deep bow toward me they acknowledged my "clapping of a single hand. . . ."

The musicians had left the podium, and while I was collecting my belongings, consisting of a cane and a little handbag, my friends and closer acquaintances from the audience slowly began to gather around me to express their pleasure at my return to the "normal" world. As I slowly made my way to the door of the music room, I heard myself being praised for walking so well that my limp was scarcely noticeable though I still wore a brace. Others inquired solicitously as to how much longer I would have to use my cane. My answer, that I really did not know but assumed it would have to be forever, left my questioners unsatisfied. They kept urging me to assume a more optimistic attitude, to give them some more detailed information as to the extent of my paralysis, and whether it would eventually go away.

No answers to these increasingly irritating questions were possible. I quickly went to the exit, waving farewell with my cane to my friends and my hosts who had accompanied me to the door. There I was met by my husband, Hans, who took my arm and carefully guided me across the thin layer of new snow that had fallen on the sidewalk. When he had placed me on the front seat of the car and seated himself, he asked, "How was the concert?" Unaccountably, I began to weep. It was one of the earlier, but by no means the only time since the onset of my illness that I broke out into seemingly unmotivated emotional spells. Initially, such spells of weeping, or even noisy sobbing, frightened and embarrassed me as much as they did my husband and my closest friends. On this occasion Hans tried to make me talk in order to find out what had caused this inordinate expression of grief. But as usual, then and later, I was incapable of speaking at all let alone of giving a rational explanation, except to admit to myself an immense grief at my permanent impairment and at the insensitivity of the human world around me as well.

The most embarrassing of my many weeping spells occurred on the occasion of a visit to Anna Freud's home in London, at 20 Maresfield Gardens in Hampstead. In this case, as in many others, at least I was able to understand my bizarre behavior even if I was incapable of explaining it to her or to the friend who had accompanied me on this visit to the distinguished lady. I initiated this visit because Anna Freud and I had several important professional milestones in common. We had both been elected in the same year as honorary fellows of the American Psychiatric Association and had also both served as Alfred P. Sloan Visiting Professors at the Menninger Foundation and Clinic in Topeka, Kansas.

My friend and I arrived at Maresfield Gardens at the appointed time of half-past four to have a cup of afternoon tea with Miss Freud. We were received by a maid, properly attired in a black uniform and white starched apron, who conducted us through a spacious hall toward a sweeping staircase. Before I had a chance to tell the maid that I was incapable of climbing the two flights of stairs, we stopped at a small door and she opened it to reveal a small elevator. The maid held it open until my friend and I had entered, and then pushed the button to take us upstairs. When the elevator stopped, the door was opened from the outside by a slim, frail-looking, elderly woman who introduced herself as Miss Freud and invited us to come into her study that was full of green plants with a strikingly tall rubber tree in the center. Otherwise, the room looked very much like the many pictures I had seen of Sigmund Freud's study, with a large desk studded with ivory and jade figurines.

In seeing the familiar-looking desk and the small woman who must have been her father's pride and joy as well as perhaps his most important disciple, I thought of the old gentleman in his eighties, dying of a malignant tumor in his jaw, having to flee from Vienna and settling in this place in London where a house was furnished to look exactly like his Viennese home. These thoughts, and the sight of the cool and distant graying lady who stood silently before me with a questioning expression, induced in me the dreadful response of a weeping spell. Evidently, to Miss Freud it was a sign of mysterious behavior, for she did not say a word until I had stopped sobbing and then she rang the bell for tea. From then on we made polite conversation about the events we shared in our lives, including my years of residence in the Berggasse while I was a medical student in Vienna. The burden of the conversation rested on me; only occasionally did she prompt me with a question or two. I sensed that she wanted to keep me talking while I was still dry-eyed, because she realized that I might break into tears again at any minute.

But now I had caught hold of myself and remained calm

so long as we were in the Maresfield Gardens house. Even when she took us downstairs to show me her father's study and his collection of exotic antiques I breathed deeply and swallowed the tears that seemed to clog my throat. Half an hour later, Miss Freud's small black poodle joined us; he took noisy exception to my cane and tried to push it away from me. This somewhat amusing incident forever dispelled the solemnity for me of the ambience of the house of the late Sigmund Freud and I took it as a signal to take leave of Miss Freud and her protective poodle and conclude my visit.

Oddly, the only living beings who seemed to comprehend the enormous sorrow expressed by my weeping without requesting an explanation were our dachshund, Wenzel, and our cat, Katinka. Every time I wept at home, they quickly climbed onto my lap and pressed their cool noses and cheeks against mine. They also seemed to enjoy lapping up my salty tears and left me only when the weeping had stopped and I had become calm once more.

From the memory of my studies in neurology of long ago, I knew that inappropriate weeping is a frequent accompaniment of some strokes, as is a tendency towards equally inappropriate laughter. I was perhaps fortunate, I told myself, not to have been fated to endure as many ill-timed spells of laughter as of weeping. It took my husband a long time and endless patience to get used to putting up with a wife weeping, yes even sobbing, in public, in restaurants, often at theater and concert performances. Worse even than that: I was sometimes overcome by these uncontrollable spells of weeping when we had guests, whose horrified reaction invariably was, "What have I said or done that hurt you?" or "Is there anything I can do to help?"

Like that earlier time when I was weeping after the chamber-music concert and incapable of stopping or explaining the cause for my noisy grief, I have since remained unable even to give an explanation, and have left dozens of friends and strangers deeply puzzled and embarrassed.

Naturally I also weep, and have wept, on such occasions that must appear sad to healthy people, as when the unveiling of the Washington War Memorial honoring the victims of the Vietnam War was shown on television. Every time I see that long black monument on the television screen with its endless rows and columns of names engraved on it, I begin to weep, as I also shed tears when I hear taps being sounded on the occasion of a military funeral or simply at the daily lowering of a flag at a military installation.

From these examples it should appear evident that my weeping is not entirely motiveless; it is, however, unrestrained and the result of facilitation—like the facilitation of other reflexes in cases of strokes, which is the result of disinhibition. To a lesser extent it is also embarrassing that I can't stop laughing where normally I would smile briefly or have a momentary giggle protracting this expression of mirth. Other reactions which I am aware as being typically due to right-brain damage, such as the fading and gradual return of my ability to identify pieces of music, I have described in another section of this book. I am fortunate in not suffering from any disturbing communication deficits, nor does neuro-ophthalmological examination reveal the existence of homonymous hemianopia (equilateral loss of vision) which is one of the most frequent left hemisensory deficits.

I am very lucky also in having retained my memory of foreign languages—including those I learned as an adult—and also including the visual memory of the ideograms of East Asian script which I have been studying for decades. I can read and write the ideograms that are familiar to me just as I could before my stroke. So far as evaluation of the permanent damage I suffered as the result of the nondominant hemisphere involvement of my stroke is concerned, I can refer mainly to my mathematical deficit, which also is mentioned elsewhere, and to my own observations of having been spared most of my intellectual and emotional functions.

The Cerebral Vascular Accident

My first social appearance at that chamber-music concert took place exactly nine months after the "cerebral vascular accident" that deprived me of the use of half of my body. This "accident," medically abbreviated as CVA, occurred three months after my husband and I had moved from the Middle West to northern California, where the university had established a new professorship for me. At the time of our move from Chicago to northern California I was barely fifty years old; we had been married for nearly thirty years. I had not yet experienced menopause, and I believed I could look forward to years of contented academic work.

I was a junior in the gymnasium (German secondary school) when I met Hans, already a doctor of jurisprudence. Although he was thirteen years my senior, we immediately enjoyed each other's company immensely. We married three years later when I was in medical school. In the thirty-two years of our marriage our happy relationship persisted and has remained a happy one to this day, in our fifty-fifth year of marriage! When we came to California, Hans and I believed I could look forward to at least a decade and a half of successful teaching and research. Hans had just concluded his career by retirement and was, perhaps, a bit apprehensive as to what his life of leisure would be in a new environment and side by side with a very busy and ambitious professional wife. Whatever his apprehensions, he soon perceived them to be entirely unfounded: Instead of spending his time in retirement, he suddenly found himself with more work than he had ever bargained for. But I must stress that the enormous workload that had so precipitously come to rest on his shoulders was entirely self-chosen and that he welcomed it, as he preferred to look after me and my many needs, including our household, rather than lose even one iota of our privacy to nursing or household personnel.

Although he had never before shown any interest in running a household, marketing, or cooking, immediately on my return from the hospital he requested that I put together shopping lists for our household needs and give him simple instructions for the cooking of uncomplicated meals. He has now long dispensed with my instructions and has become a skillful cook, able to prepare our simple, low-calorie meals quickly and without any fuss. Whereas at the beginning of his householding career he would generally ask me what I wanted to eat so that he could shop accordingly, he now makes his own decisions according to his own taste and skill. He rarely permits me to participate in his cooking rituals, as he does not wish me to tire myself by standing at the kitchen counter or the stove. The one exception is in the preparation of scrambled eggs which he maintains I can cook better than anyone else. But since we do not eat that dish very often, I have little opportunity to practice my cooking skills and, odd as it may appear, I find that I miss this activity which had occupied me for three decades.

Moreover, from the very moment of the onset of my paralysis it had been Hans's fervent wish that I shouldn't lose any time by learning tiring one-handed skills, but that I should rather resume the scholarly and professional life I had led prior to my stroke. In fact, when I first realized that I had lost the use of one hand—probably permanently—and broke into one of my earliest spells of uncontrolled weeping, it had been Hans who spent his days and nights in the hospital at my bedside, who said, "Formerly you had two hands, now you have three, because you also have my two hands to assist the one that is left to you." And so it has remained.

3
The Event: Functions Lost and Retained

And now that I have said so much about the relatively youthful age at which I suffered my stroke, I think it is time to tell what preceded it and how it happened.

It simply happened on March 28, 1964, Saturday morning of that Easter weekend. The extraordinary aspect of this date is that exactly one year earlier, March 28, 1963, I had suffered another major accident that also involved my left leg. That earlier accident occurred in Honolulu, where I stopped on a lecture trip around the world to give a speech at the University of Hawaii on the occasion of the inauguration of the university's new president. My lecture was formal, well attended, and well received. In the evening a dinner party was arranged in honor of the new president and the speaker. The lively conversation dealt with various aspects of oriental medicine, whose history had long been one of my major topics of research. One of the dinner guests, a middle-aged Chinese woman, related that her mother knew of a very effective local analgesic that was part of the old Chinese materia medica. It consisted of eucalyptus leaves steeped in an alcoholic liquid, in whiskey for instance, a mixture that was to be applied to the injured and painful area, which would then cease hurting almost immediately. With some amusement and disbelief we discussed the respective merits of the various types of whiskeys. Finally, we concluded this topic of conversation with an expression of devout hope that none of us would require a strong topical analgesic in the near future.

Following Hawaiian custom, the dinner party ended early; moreover, I had to pack my suitcases and prepare myself for an early flight to Japan on the following morning. So I rose and thanked my hosts and the newly inaugurated university president for their hospitality and the stimulating evening. My host offered to see me to his car and drive me to the hotel. When we stepped outside, we noticed that a light rain had begun to fall and had covered the stone steps of his house with a thin film of moisture. Unprepared for the slipperiness of wet stairs, I began to descend, and after the second or third step I slipped and fell onto the sidewalk. In hitting the flagstones of the sidewalk, I felt an acute pain in my left ankle at the same time that I heard a high, cracking sound. I knew one of my anklebones was broken and asked my host to take me to the emergency room of Queen's Hospital so that I could have the fracture set.

During the short ride to the hospital, I thought of the many telegrams and letters I would have to send to call off my lecture engagements in Tokyo, Taipeh, Hong Kong, Athens, Vienna, Rome, Munich, and Bonn. Naturally, my friends and colleagues in Honolulu were chagrined at my mishap in their radiantly beautiful city. An orthopedist was called and came shortly after my arrival in the hospital. He ordered an x-ray, and soon was able to diagnose a spiral fracture of the left fibula. He applied a knee-high cast that permitted me to walk carefully for short distances, so that my stay at the hospital was limited largely to having breakfast and spending the nights in my room. For lunch and dinner I was usually taken out by some of the many friends and acquaintances I had met in the course of my frequent visits in Hawaii.

During the brief period that I wore that cast I became accustomed to walking with a cane, so it seemed quite natural to me to do so when, a year later, I again became dependent upon the support of a cane. On the occasion of that earlier accident in Honolulu I received my first instructions from a physical therapist on how to use an extraneous support, such as a crutch or a cane. I learned that it is necessary to carry the cane in the hand of the uninjured side, a method that was again applicable a year later when my hemiplegia (paralysis of one side of the body) did not leave me a choice as to which hand I was to use to carry my cane. I also learned in Honolulu that in negotiating stairs exact rules must be followed: in walking upstairs the uninjured foot goes first, whereas in walking downstairs the injured leg precedes. That all these rules should become general knowledge must be clear to an observant moviegoer or television watcher, where many actors, playing the parts of injured soldiers or civilians, wrongly support themselves with canes or crutches on the damaged side.

In Honolulu my orthopedist advised me to extend my stay beyond the three days I had booked originally. He also suggested that I delay my long and strenuous lecture trip that was to have taken me through much of east Asia and most of central Europe.

Naturally, I had to cancel my flight reservation to Tokyo and my subsequent flights to all the other cities where I was to have lectured. Two days later, in the morning, I was advised that two Japanese gentlemen were at the hospital to call on me. Their calling cards indicated that they were the chief representatives of Japan Airlines in Honolulu and the Japanese consul general. They arrived formally dressed in black suits and carried a large bouquet of orchids. They had come to express their sympathy over my lost trip to the Orient. Like everyone else they expressed the hope that another occasion would arise for me to travel around the world. As it happened, "the other occasion" never arose and the trip around the world—even though the lecture invitations arrived—fell victim to my "accident" a year later.

Instead of taking a glorious trip around the world, I decided to return home to Chicago where my arrival at O'Hare Airport in a wheelchair, with my leg in a cast, seemed like a pitiful anticlimax. Five weeks after the fracture I went to the orthopedic clinic at the university and had an x-ray taken which revealed a satisfactory callus formation in my fractured fibula; two weeks later my cast could be removed and the first accident forgotten. The coincidence of both accidents, the fracture and the stroke, happening on March 28, has occupied my thoughts a great deal. Was that date an anniversary of an earlier disaster? I never found an answer to this question.

On Saturday morning of March 28, 1964, I had awakened a bit too early for a holiday weekend and put myself back to sleep, from which I awakened half an hour later. As I usually did once a month, I decided to palpate my breasts as a precautionary measure, in order to discover whether I had any nodules or irregularities and to avoid previously unnoticed development of a possible malignant growth. I palpated thoroughly with my right hand, first feeling my left breast and axilla. After completing that part of the examination I tried to lift my left arm in order to palpate my right breast. To my utter bafflement I found myself unable to do so. Not even a finger could I move. Gradually it dawned on me that I was now experiencing the results of some mysterious symptoms I had been noticing for more than a month. To confirm or test my suspicion of the nature of the sudden paralysis, I used my right arm to make myself sit up on the edge of the bed. I had scarcely accomplished this, when I fell over on my left side, unable to guard myself with my left hand. When I tried to get up to walk to the bathroom I realized that my left leg and foot were playing the same game with me as my arm and hand. Evidently, I thought, a stroke had afflicted the entire left side. I decided to stop coping with this phenomenon myself and to call my husband. Before doing so I silently rehearsed his name, then I called it aloud. The result was an unattractive croaking sound which brought him to my bedside almost immediately.

"What's the matter?" he said with some anxiety. "I cannot speak very well," I replied, "I have dysarthria." This last word is not part of our daily domestic vocabulary; besides, it was pronounced so indistinctly that he had no idea what I was trying to say. So he said, "Why don't you sit up and come for breakfast? I just made it." As best I could I said, "I cannot sit up; my left side is paralyzed." This time, my words came out almost fluently and the hoarse sound had left my voice. We decided that it seemed appropriate to call a physician.

This was easier said than done. As newcomers to the region where we had been living for scarcely more than two months we were medical orphans, and had no idea whom to call. Even though my work as a professor of medical history was conducted in a university hospital, it had not occurred to me to make contact with any physician who would serve as a family doctor. To be sure, the peculiar symptoms I had been experiencing during the last six weeks would have been reason enough to see a doctor; instead, I kept on reading about them in the medical literature and felt that they simply represented symptoms of a transitory disturbance, not serious enough to merit much fuss and bother. Now that the disaster had struck and I found myself the victim of hemiplegia, I remembered a recent dinner party where we had met a neurologist who seemed appropriate for our present situation. I succeeded in recalling his name and pronouncing it clearly enough so that my husband could find it in the telephone book. Since it was a Saturday morning he happened to be home and free to come to the phone. He promised to come to our house right away, although a little later he would have to catch a plane and fly to the East Coast for an important meeting which was to begin the day after Easter.

He arrived in almost half an hour equipped with reflex hammer, needles, and his own mental diagnostic equipment that made it evident to him, as I had suspected, that I suffered a cerebral vascular accident and should be hospitalized right away. No one in the world can imagine how grateful I was to hear the expression "cerebral vascular accident." It seemed such an elegantly youthful affliction as compared to "stroke," which I had used all along in my private conversation with myself. A stroke denoted a drab condition of elderly, if not to say, old, patients, and there wasn't anything really scientific about it. But CVA had that learned elegance and—innocent as I was at that time— suggested a matter of impermanence.

Soon after he had completed his preliminary examination the ambulance arrived and took me across that beautiful bridge to one of the big university hospitals. I was much too drowsy to be fully aware of the length of the ambulance ride, but I knew that the brief examination had not provided a definitive diagnosis and that sinister though a stroke, or even CVA, might sound, there were alternative and even worse possibilities of what might have happened in my brain. So I kept on testing the impairments, and the faculties I had retained; I tried to move my left arm and hand or wiggle my left toes, both without any success. Evidently, I realized, the damage must be located in the right side of my brain, hence it seemed reasonable that I had retained my faculty of speech and visual memory. To test the validity of this reasoning, I began to count to ten in all the languages known to me. In pronouncing the words for the numbers, I also visualized their spelling or the ideograms that represented them. The ambulance driver and orderly who heard me murmur to myself exchanged amused and knowing glances.

4
The Hospital: Tender, Loving Care?

Having completed my full linguistic repertoire to my own satisfaction, I fell asleep. I only woke up again after I had been placed in my hospital bed and a nurse was busy taking my blood pressure over and over again. This was repeated so often that the tightness of the cuff of the sphygmomanometer on my right arm began to irritate and give me a feeling of soreness on my arm. Besides, I wanted to be left alone to sleep. When I woke there were several people in my room, a couple of nurses and a youthful-looking man in a white coat whom I took to be the neurologist sent by the physician who had examined me at home. The new neurologist approached my bed; seeing that I was awake he introduced himself as Dr. Martin Klein who would from now on have the pleasure of taking care of me. He suggested that we be left alone and gestured for the nurses and residents to leave the room.

On this first moment of awareness in my hospital room an amusing incident took place—at least it seemed amusing to me. Among the nurses and residents who had been sent away by Dr. Klein there was one young man with marked oriental features which I interpreted to be Japanese. In order to check whether this guess was correct, I asked him, in what I assumed to be his native language, whether he had come from Japan and what his name was. Before he had time to recover from his astonishment at being addressed in his own language and reply, Dr. Klein interrupted our incompleted communication and said, "It seems that the patient is more confused than we had at first assumed, as her communication is quite disordered." The young Japanese physician smiled and replied with a marked Japanese accent, "I am afraid you are mistaken, Dr. 'Kurain.' Dr. Veith spoke in faultless Japanese." With this reply he bowed and left Dr. Klein speechless with surprise and departed from the room. To my regret, I never saw the young Japanese doctor again and I gathered that he had been transferred for duty in another wing of the neurological floor of the hospital.

After having gone through the routine of a neurological physical examination similar to the one I had experienced at home, Dr. Klein inquired into the history of my illness and the symptoms that might have preceded my accident. It so happened that I had been quite conscious of a number of physical changes that had been occurring in the past two months, in fact, more or less since I moved to the new university. The most drastic change I noted was an overwhelming migraine involving the right side of my head. It had not responded to any analgesics available to me. Because I have long been sensitive to aspirin, I had to resort to fifteen milligrams of codeine left over from an earlier painful condition. But not even the codeine freed me completely from pain for more than an hour. Although I would fall asleep with a feeling that the pain of the headache had abated, I generally would wake up some few hours later with renewed throbbing in the right side of my head and face.

Having suffered from occasional bouts of migraine throughout my life and never having elicited any particular interest for this affliction in any of my colleagues or family doctors, I had given little thought to finding a physician who would, in any case, probably have told me that there was little to be done against migraine except taking analgesics or one of the ergot products which, in turn, might have their own disagreeable side effects. Having completed this hypothetical conversation with the nonexisting physicians, I decided to try my luck with one or two of the six remaining pills of a bottle of Ergotrate that had been prescribed to me on an earlier occasion of migraine.

All this I conveyed to Dr. Klein. He interrupted me from time to time requesting that I describe the nature of my "headache." I was aware that he used the word headache rather than migraine in a somewhat condescending fashion and then urged me to describe further symptoms. Irritated by his uninvited switch in terminology I asked him whether he knew the etymology of the word "migraine," a question he impatiently tried to circumvent by saying that most patients could not tell the difference. Whereupon I informed him in my own somewhat condescending fashion that migraine was derived from the Latin *hemicrania*, and that, in turn, from the Greek *hemi kranion*, meaning literally "half of the skull." Dr. Klein listened to this somewhat pedantic explanation with obvious boredom and displeasure and then asked me again whether that pain in one side of the head was accompanied by other unusual symptoms. "Yes, it was," I admitted and proceeded to explain that I had experienced repeated bouts of scintillating scotoma which came upon me without prior warning.

I considered it unnecessary to explain to him, the neurologist, what scintillating scotomas were, and how frightening the crystalline glitter is that suddenly occupies the center of one's field of vision and leaves the victim nearly blind. I had fallen prey to these distressing symptoms at irregular intervals, sometimes when I was driving my car in the bright light of the afternoon sun. It left me feeling greatly handicapped in coping with the traffic whether it was oncoming or moving in my own direction. As a rule, these spells of near-blindness lasted between fifteen and twenty minutes. It is difficult to describe the relief when my sight returned to normal as suddenly as it had disappeared. Fortunately and miraculously, I never suffered an accident during these exceedingly vulnerable periods of near-blindness.

As a sequel to my mentioning the origin of hemicrania and Dr. Klein's ironic reply, he now inquired whether I would again like to offer an etymological explanation for scintillating scotomas. I knew then that I had lost most of his empathy and decided to express myself in simple terms to keep me in the category of a patient that would not pose a challenge to the physician. Unfortunately, there was a third symptom for which I could not offer such a simple lay expression. I told him I had been experiencing olfactory hallucinations for at least two months prior to my stroke. The illusory scent that accompanied me day and night was that of ripe limes. This was a most pleasant odor even though I knew it was totally imaginary as our house was surrounded by lemon and orange trees, simultaneously in bloom and fruit, and there was not a single lime tree in sight.

Dr. Klein, who had been silently taking notes throughout my narrative, looked up coolly and said: "Migraine—oh, pardon me, hemicrania—scintillating scotoma, and olfactory hallucinations, an interesting combination and quite telling of a forthcoming stroke." "But is it a stroke?" I interrupted his musings, evidently to his displeasure, for he replied, "You might have let me finish my sentence. There were a number of further questions I wanted to ask you. Since you've been so aware of your abnormal symptoms, didn't it occur to you that you might better see a physician?" I nodded in full agreement and admitted that now that things had turned out the way they had, I clearly had chosen to have a "fool for a doctor"—indicating myself.

My failure to try to establish contact with an internist or a neurologist when I began having migraines and scintillating scotomas was due not so much to an unforgivable indifference or disbelief in the severity of the symptoms, but to an unfortunate coincidence of my own research and the literature given to me by Dr. Hammerman of the clinical faculty of the Department of Ophthalmology. He described the histories of a number of patients suffering from various forms of migraine and scintillating scotoma, most of whom were women. From the totality of his observations the physician concluded that these disturbances undoubtedly were symptoms of hysterical personality.

Dr. Hammerman's writings were by no means the first I had read that associated visual disturbances and migraine with certain aspects of hysteria. This subject was of particular interest to me because I was, at the time, at work on a fairly ambitious book on the history of hysteria. In fact, most of my reading in the years before I moved to California had been associated with aspects of hysteria. No wonder I was inclined to assume that my own visual disturbances, together with those attacks of migraine, were indications that I had fallen victim to the disease of my studies* and that there was little point in consulting a physician.

When I found one side of myself completely paralyzed, I felt certain that I was a case in line with my researches

---

*Ilza Veith, "Blinders of the Mind: Historical Reflections on Functional Impairments of Vision." *Bulletin of the History of Medicine*, vol. 48, Winter 1974.

on hysteria.* Initially, I deluded myself that if I admitted the hysterical nature of my hemiplegia to myself and others, it would simply go away. Such was the solution derived from the venerable sources of my research on the history of hysteria. Unfortunately, my attempts at autosuggestion did not measure up to the expertise of the great doctors of the past who were more skillful and convincing in the treatment of their impaired patients than I was.

"In that case," Dr. Klein continued, "I assume there is little point in asking you about the history of your blood pressure, which is low now." "But then," I volunteered, "I no longer have any of the other symptoms, migraine or scotoma, nor olfactory hallucinations." Nevertheless, Dr. Klein suggested that I should go through all the necessary diagnostic procedures to rule out whatever diagnosis did not apply, and to find out what kind of a stroke I had.

In contrast to the assumption of most people that all strokes are more or less alike, a stroke is not just a stroke; there are subtle differences between the various causes of the sudden paralysis. Strokes have in common only that this paralysis usually reflects an abnormality in the arteries supplying blood to the brain, caused by either a thrombosis or an embolism and resulting in an occlusion or the rupture of a dilated artery, an aneurysm, followed by a hemorrhage.

In my case it was uncertain which one it had been, a thrombosis or a ruptured aneurysm, or even a silent tumor, which might have caused the sudden paralysis. It seemed, however, in the first few days that my affliction was not regarded as a fait accompli that would simply keep me in my present state of impairment, but that there was a possibility of an extension or worsening of my state. I believed

---

*Veith, *History of Hysteria: The History of a Disease* (Chicago: The University of Chicago Press, 1965).

it was for this reason that my blood pressure was measured so frequently and that I was instructed to remain as quiet as possible.

Because Hans was aware of the continued precariousness of the state of my health, he persisted in his steady presence in my hospital room, day and night, so as not to miss a possible worsening of my condition. Naturally, he never told me of the reason for his constant presence there, nor of his great concern for my recovery. Every time I was served one of my meager meals I realized that he had not yet eaten anything, and only after repeated urging on my part did he leave briefly for what I assumed was a hasty and extremely modest lunch or supper in the hospital cafeteria. Although he was lean to start with, he lost all the weight that I was supposed to lose on my careful low-calorie diet.

Thus he was in my room when, about three days after the dreadful event and my hospitalization, I was informed that I would have to have a lumbar puncture (also known as a spinal tap), a procedure by which a small amount of fluid is withdrawn from the spinal canal to find out whether it contained any trace of blood. The physician who was to do this procedure was young, still a resident, and very pleasant. He introduced himself as Dr. Adriani and requested that I lie on my right side with my knees drawn up as high as possible, "in the fetal position, so to speak," as he said. I was somewhat apprehensive about the after-effects of this procedure, as I had heard that if it were done too fast or the needle withdrawn too rapidly it could be followed by a severe headache. As it was, I did not feel the needle enter my spine nor be withdrawn, nor did I get a headache later. In fact, I felt well, apart from the pain in my paralyzed and increasingly contracted left limbs. And for that reason I needed continued rest and freedom from excitement.

Nevertheless there still remained some uncertainty as to the exact location of the cerebral lesion. Further tests were planned. Dr. Klein did not permit me to have any visitors or telephone calls, though my speech had become entirely fluent and my voice had lost its rasping quality, because he thought that visitors would excite me too much. Instead, he went through the daily routine of holding out his hand and asking me to squeeze his fingers with my left (paralyzed) hand. This futile exercise, which was intended to elicit signs of spontaneous recovery, annoyed me very much because it followed my own daily self-examination which I carried out every morning immediately on waking. In fact, it took weeks before I was made to realize that the paralysis of my left arm and hand was complete and probably irreversible. This happened after the major neurological examinations had been completed and I was deemed fit enough to undergo physiotherapy.

My supervised exercises began after I had spent a week in the hospital and had undergone a skull x-ray and an electroencephalogram (EEG) as well as a radioisotope brain scan (following an intravenous injection). In the clinical summary of my case, the radioisotope scan was reported as normal. The electroencephalogram was "abnormal," as it showed "a slowing over the right temporoparietal areas, suggesting injury in that area." A right carotid angiogram showed marked narrowing in the internal carotid artery over a very short segment. There was also probable occlusion of branches of the middle cerebral artery.

It was my misfortune to have become ill a decade too early, for in 1964 a brain scan meant my lying prone in an uncomfortable position on a flat pad on the floor, my head supported by a stiffened foam-rubber wedge while the x-ray machine slid back and forth close to my forehead. In the many years since then great improvements have been made in the accurate diagnosis of certain diseases of the brain by the invention of computerized axial tomography, now popularly known as the CAT scanner. For reasons entirely unrelated to my stroke, I had an occasion later on to become acquainted with this sophisticated diagnostic tool as well, and was agreeably surprised by the relative comfort that the CAT scanner offered the patient compared to the older, nuclear brain scan. I was amused, however, by its shape, which resembled a wooden tunnel with a narrow entrance from which protruded a long, narrow board—somewhat like an ironing board. On this board the patient rests, held secure with leather bandages. Then board and patient are pushed into the tunnel of the scanner a little like a baker pushing his loaves of bread into the oven. After about an hour, during which the circular scanner rotates around the body in the tunnel, the patient is drawn out on his board, ready to be diagnosed from the many x-ray pictures the scanner has taken.

But the nuclear brain scan was all that was available at the time I was stricken and again, a little later, when I fell on my head owing to the carelessness and inexperience of a student nurse. The nurse left me standing, unsupported, in my room while she responded to a summons from outside. This happened so soon after my stroke that I had not yet developed any sense of balance and was simply unable to stand on my one good leg.

Brain Scan and the Mirage of Recovery

The first radionuclear brain-scan examination I experienced was as unpleasant and uncomfortable as most traditional x-ray examinations tend to be. At any rate, for some time I mistakenly associated a coincidental beneficial event with this brain scan: On my return to my room from the x-ray department I went through my frequent routine of trying to move each of my left extremities, fingers, leg, and toes—all of which had been totally paralyzed since the "accident"—and to my great amazement I suddenly found that I could move my left hip and knee at will, but not my toes, my arm, or my fingers. That will come too, I thought. When Dr. Klein appeared for his daily visit soon after the scan I called his attention to my newly discovered ability to move my leg and told him I thought I might begin to walk very soon. He denied this and said it was necessary to complete my neurological examination first: moreover, he added, I would be needing a leg brace to steady my leg and ankle.

For the next major neurological examination, the neurologist said, I would have to give my written consent, for which a resident would visit me in the evening with the appropriate forms. Upon my inquiry into the nature of this examination Dr. Klein said casually that it was to be another radiological examination, known as a "carotid angiogram." When I asked what its exact purpose was and whether it was unpleasant, he replied that owing to the contrast medium that was to be injected into the carotid artery, I would experience a slight feeling of warmth in my head. Its purpose was to pinpoint the exact location of my cerebral vascular accident. The day after the angiogram, I was to be fitted for a leg brace and, if the physical therapy department happened to have a spare brace, "we" could begin with the physical therapy and I might begin to learn to walk.

As usual, when the neurologist ended his visit and left the room, I fell asleep. I did not even come fully awake when my husband came in and sat down in the reclining chair with which my room was equipped. Thanks to the remarkable thoughtfulness on the part of the hospital and administration, he was able to make up in part for the many sleepless nights he had spent in my hospital room, worrying about my uncertain future.

In the evening I was awakened at dusk by a young physician, whom I took to be the resident, who had come to request that I sign the form permitting the angiogram procedure. Routinely I asked that the headpiece of my bed be cranked up so that I could give my signature in a semiupright position.

I also had to ask the resident to hold the paper onto the clipboard with both hands because the form would move if I were to try to sign it without such stabilization. My observation that it is impossible to write on any paper, stationery, or postcard without a second hand holding it steady, laid the foundation of my vast collection of paperweights with which I can counterbalance the pages upon which I am writing. Only one of my many friends who sent me presents—most of which were far from useful—sent a magnificent paperweight, a Steuben glass owl, which I have continued to use and treasure ever since it came to me some eighteen years ago.

The Horror of the Carotid Angiogram

At any rate, I quickly (much too quickly, I later realized) read through the form requesting my permission to submit to the carotid angiogram and found that it scarcely differed from previous forms I had signed for medical, surgical, and radiological manipulations. There was no special paragraph warning of the possible danger of side effects, nor of the incredible pain and discomfort I was to experience during the procedure. I signed the form as best I could and the resident left me with the customary, "Take care," a suggestion of leave-taking used by everyone on the hospital staff which always left me baffled. What should I take care of? There was nothing I could have done to take care to avoid my cerebral vascular accident or any other diffi-

The Hospital: Tender, Loving Care?

culty I had to or was going to encounter in my life. I replied by saying good night to the resident and fell asleep right away.

At dawn on the following morning I was awakened by a nurse and an orderly pushing a gurney into my room. With great skill I was transferred from my bed onto the gurney and immediately wheeled into the elevator that took me to the x-ray department. Here I was awaited by the radiologist who specialized in making carotid angiograms. He looked at me briefly and, with a short greeting, took hold of a fairly large syringe that he filled with a colorless fluid. Then he motioned me to lie back on the gurney, onto which my arms and legs were fastened with wide straps of cloth. Without any further words he positioned the needle of the syringe upon the carotid artery on the right side of my neck and, a second later, without an anesthetic or even a sedative or at least a warning of the forthcoming pain, he plunged the needle of the syringe into my neck. This extremely painful procedure caused me to wince, for which I was scolded by the radiologist, who said sternly, "And now don't wince and don't moan and don't move even an inch." Immediately afterwards he pushed the plunger into the syringe, and again I moaned. I also understood what my neurologist meant when he said I would feel a "little warmth" in my head. I did not feel warm, I felt as though my brain were on fire. The first injection was followed by a second and third, during each of which I was told not to moan. The repeated pain was incredibly severe, as was the frightening experience of believing that my head was on fire and ready to explode.

After the fourth injection of the radiopaque dye the radiologist said, "That's it," and motioned a nurse and orderly to take hold of my gurney and return me to my room. By the time I returned it was "dinnertime," as lunch was described by the dietician who served our meals on the minute. I also found my husband, whom I welcomed with my no longer unusual stream of tears, waiting for me. I still remembered the fiery injection into my head and began to tremble all over. As usual when I was weeping I was unable to speak and could not answer my husband when he asked me about the test I had just undergone. So ravaged did I feel after the angiogram that I remained incapable of talking about it for several days. In later years I heard from fellow-sufferers of this traumatic procedure that they had been sedated, some even anesthetized, prior to the angiogram and had not felt it as painfully humiliating as I did.

In the course of my stay at the hospital my windowsill became filled to overflow with daily gifts of flowers from local friends and from those all over the country who had heard about my illness. The hospital volunteers, a great number of very gentle women all of whom seemed to look alike in their gray-and-white speckled uniforms, took special pleasure in taking care of my flowers and watering them early in the morning. So early, in fact, that they usually came into my room when I was still fast asleep, a sleep for which I had fought a hard battle, since I was not allowed any sedatives or sleeping pills, because they might obscure the picture of my illness and alter the symptoms. Hence, I was always very irritated when the "gray lady" of the day made her appearance asking, "And how are we today?"

My sleeping habits during my hospital stay may seem strange and contradictory. During the daytime, when I was alone in the room except for my husband's quiet presence, I felt sleepy all day long and fell asleep rapidly and often. At night, on the other hand, although I was tired—too tired to read—I was so beset by unhappiness over my illness that I found my thoughts occupied with plans and questions about the future, or rather with profound worries about my professional future, which had looked so promising and happy a few months earlier when we moved to California.

Another complication arose from my hemiplegia. I had not anticipated this complication, nor had the friends who sent me presents. It was generally known that I had always been an avid reader. So it was assumed that now that I was hospitalized, with more "time on my hands" (a pun made by several people, perhaps unintentionally) than I needed, I could do all the reading I wanted. So they sent me books; and since they were generous people and aimed to make me lasting presents, they sent me books in hard covers. Unfortunately, I was unable to hold hard-cover books in bed with one hand. So I sent out requests for paperbacks, which I could manage single-handed provided they were not too thick and heavy. I was unable to turn pages in magazines and newspapers that were brought to me in large quantities. Although I love to read and, indeed, had "all that time on my hands," I much preferred to sleep and, eventually, I often did for at least part of the night.

Thus, with the best of intentions, the "gray ladies" disrupted my sleep. In addition to the watering can, the gray lady invariably carried a stack of newspapers and asked me whether I wished to buy one. Not just once, but every day during my hospital stay I would have to explain to the benevolent volunteer that: a) I did not wish to be awakened from my hard-earned sleep with the trivia she had to dispense; and b) I was unable to handle and read a newspaper, as it was impossible for me to hold it up and turn the pages with one hand; so would she please refrain from now on from offering me this useless entertainment. Each gray lady listened to me with a mild expression, possibly not comprehending the reason for my annoyance. Sometimes one of the women would tell me that she would be able to read a newspaper easily with one hand. Whereupon I grumpily replied, "Well, show me; but regardless of what you can do with a newspaper, don't offer me one for sale when I am still fast asleep—and please tell your colleagues not to bother me so early in the morning." I must have sounded so unfriendly, so totally ungrateful for the efforts they were making, that they assumed I had suffered an emotional disturbance.

Gradually I came to realize that my irritated reaction to the kind "gray ladies" had been evolving ever since I had been hospitalized. In thinking about this unfortunate change in my formerly cheerful personality, I began to suspect that it resulted from resentment at my helplessness and the ever-increasing pain due to the contractures of my paralyzed limbs. Later on, when I was allowed to receive visitors, I frequently found myself offended by the ignorance in the opinions offered generously by my nonmedical acquaintances. Thus when told over and over again that, after all, I was well off, inasmuch as my left paralyzed side was unable to perceive pain, I heard myself snarl at the kindly souls who had come with bunches of flowers and boxes of sweets to the uninviting corridors of the hospital, meaning so well when they tried to comfort me with their untutored opinions. I could almost read their minds when—offended by my ungracious reaction to their well-meaning chatter—they decided not to expose themselves again unnecessarily to my ill humor and obvious depression.

The gray lady, however, did not feel helpless in the face of my unfriendly reception of her kindliness. She considered it to be the signs of an acute depression and passed on this observation to the medical staff. A few days later the door opened and a slight, youthful-looking man in a white doctor's coat came into my room and took a chair beside my bed. He took my right hand, said good morning, and introduced himself as a psychiatric resident, Dr. Mittenwald. Although I was very much amused by this extremely appropriate name for a psychiatrist, I was in no mood to have a psychiatric consultation which I had not initiated. I told this to Dr. Mittenwald and asked him to leave my room as I knew my depression was caused by concrete reasons and that no psychiatrist could help me unless he could work a miracle and cure my hemiplegia. The psychiatrist realized that I was entirely determined in my rejection of his services and left my room with an unhappy face, wishing me the best of luck with the inevitable, "Take care."

By the time I had gotten rid of the psychiatrist I had overcome most of the physical insult and the traumatic memory of the angiogram and looked at the mountain of mail that had accumulated on my bedside table. It contained one of the many medical journals I received without subscribing, sustaining itself from the masses of drug- and other medicine-related advertisements; it belonged to that category of many medical journals known as "throwaways." In looking through the table of contents of this most recently arrived journal, I found it contained an article on carotid angiograms by two of the leading Chicago neuroscientists. Naturally, I began to read it right away and found that it judged the use of arteriograms unsuitable as a diagnostic measure in the confirmation of a CVA. The reason given for rejecting the procedure was the danger of engendering additional paralyses and the extreme discomfort of the procedure.

In spite of my short, and far from polite, treatment of Dr. Mittenwald, I was quite aware of my profound depression which worsened with every day. I knew that after my return from the hospital I would eventually consider consulting a psychiatrist. But the more I thought about it, the more I realized that since my depression was caused solely by my physical defects, it could scarcely be cured by a few hours conversation in a psychiatrist's office.

Much later, after my return from the hospital when I was still as handicapped as I had been since the onset of my stroke, I felt I should test the validity of the opinion I had formed about the ineffectiveness of psychotherapy in my case. So I spent a few hours with two psychiatrists, one after the other. Apart from the generous use of the contents of several large boxes of Kleenex to dry my ever-flowing tears, I soon realized that I was not deriving much definitive benefit from this conversational therapy, nor did I derive any help from the mood-elevating medication that was prescribed for me. Yet there was one fairly important change in my emotional state that evolved during the several hours of speaking with the psychiatrists; namely, that I no longer spoke of wanting to take refuge in suicide. In fact, after having talked about it repeatedly, I became certain that I did not really wish to end my life. For after all, paralyzed or not, I still enjoyed being alive. Moreover, I was not certain whether I would be able to find an absolutely reliable way of committing suicide. I knew what it meant to be half-alive in being hemiplegic.

Having regained a considerable degree of rationality and even serenity, I decided to end my therapy and to give myself to the enjoyment of being alive and, especially, to being enveloped by my husband's warmth and comfort. Even today, after more than twenty-two years of being an invalid, there always is in the back of my mind the solace of the existence of a way out whenever I should reach the point of no longer being able to bear my permanent handicap, the pain of contractures, and my dependence upon the goodwill and helpfulness of others. But while the thought exists, I know that I shall not succumb to it.

Physical Therapy: To Stand on Both Feet

On the morning following his visit, I retained only the amused memory of the helpless Dr. Mittenwald from my previous day of pain, discomfort, and depression. By now I was thoroughly willing to try my luck with physiotherapy when the messenger arrived with the appropriate wheelchair. The room for physical therapy was in the basement of the hospital; it was large and quiet, laid out with numerous thick mattresses, and furnished with several horizontal bars. The thick mattresses, or rather heavy pads, were softly upholstered and served as support for physical exercises. At first, I was to attempt to sit on the pad for a session of "passive resistive exercises." It began by the therapist instructing me to shrug my shoulders. This seemed such a simple task to me that I was amazed that I had only one shoulder to shrug: my right shoulder. It hadn't occurred to me that my left shoulder had joined the strike of the left half of my body. Only when I supported my left elbow and pushed my arm upwards could I achieve a shrugging motion. It was only after this first physical therapy session that I subsequently became aware of how important it is for interpersonal communication to be able to shrug one's shoulder. This inability deprives me of an important mode of expressing myself.

Following the shoulder-shrugging exercise, which I was to repeat every day from then on, other passive resistive exercises were undertaken with the intention of strengthening my arms and legs. Among these the most important are the "range-of-motion" exercises, which should be performed on the paralyzed extremities every day. Range-of-motion exercises are important because they help maintain the length of the muscles and the flexibility of the joints. With the onset of a stroke, the range of motion of the shoulder joint is abruptly reduced to a minimum. When this occurs, even the attempt at range-of-motion exercises becomes excruciatingly painful and can be regained only with endless, patient practice and occasional injections with Xylocaine and cortisone. The exercises on the thick mattress lasted about thirty minutes and, in concluding it, the therapist suggested that I try changing my position without her help, or that I at least try turning over from one side to the other. In succeeding in these strenuous exercises I felt truly victorious. The therapist suggested that I repeat those exercises that I could do by myself at least once a day and I have done this faithfully for twenty-two years.

In addition to the routine I had learned at the hospital and have continued at home, I have extended my repertoire with further exercises which I carry out every night in bed before going to sleep. These are sit-up exercises. Having begun with ten sit-ups, I have gradually extended the number to thirty sit-ups. This exercise is not only strenuous, but frankly it is also boring, and to create a temporary diversion I have developed the habit of counting to ten in three different languages. Usually I begin with Japanese numbers and then follow with Chinese numbers. Sometimes, I realize that I have skipped a number and lose track of my efforts. My third series of sit-ups is usually counted in French, which is so familiar to me that I never skip any numbers. Since my internist considers strenuous and extended exercise very important for my health, I try to do the sit-ups as slowly as possible, so as to strengthen my abdominal muscles, but rarely can I extend this session much beyond twenty minutes.

After the mattress exercises in the physical-therapy room, the therapist helped me put on my heavy, large, flat shoes, which had meanwhile been delivered from the orthopedic shoe store. To the left shoe she attached a long heavy metal brace, explaining which button I had to press to bend the knee joint of the brace and press again to straighten it out. She helped me stand up and, putting a heavy orthopedic cane in my right hand, suggested that I begin to walk. To my amazement I found myself far from able to take a step on my own, losing my balance toward the paralyzed left side the moment I was standing upright.

But by walking behind me and guiding me with her hands on my hips, the therapist led me towards the parallel horizontal bars; placing me between them, she suggested that I hold on to the right-hand bar and slowly walk along it.

In the very same narrow confines I met another woman, wearing a similar brace and cane and trying to walk along the gymnastic apparatus. In contrast to me, however, she was able to guide herself on both bars with both hands even though her left leg was as paralyzed as mine. She was a heavy-set, friendly woman, and I began to talk with her about her illness and progress to recovery. She told me that her name was Mrs. Kitts and that she had suffered a stroke two years earlier. Her left arm and hand had also been totally paralyzed but then, suddenly, after a year and a half, she regained movement in that extremity. The reason for her delay in learning to walk was that soon after her CVA she had fallen and broken her left hip, which made it impossible for her to wear a brace or to bear her weight on that leg for six months. In listening to her I became determined to do everything I could to avoid falling so as not to suffer a fracture. So far, I have succeeded in keeping this promise to myself. But to my dismay I was not going to be able, like Mrs. Kitts, to regain movement in my left arm even though I had convinced myself that this would also happen to me in a year and a half. In fact, I was frightened at the prospect of having to wait that long in my half-paralyzed state and said so to the physical therapist who was supervising my awkward attempts at walking along those horizontal bars. At first the therapist listened to me without response; when I repeated my statement that I could not possibly bear to wait for more than a year to use my left arm again, she said briefly and harshly: "Don't worry, you won't ever use it again, so don't bother about that year and a half."

With these words she dismissed her class of two and sent

us back upstairs to our rooms. When I arrived I found my husband and the neurologist, neither one particularly astonished to see me in tears. "What's the reason for the tears today?" the neurologist asked, even though he knew that I would not be able to answer immediately. Eventually, I collected myself and told him and my husband that I had just been informed by the physiotherapist that I would remain paralyzed forever. The neurologist looked at me with scarcely concealed amusement and said, "What else did you expect?"

I told him of Mrs. Kitts's miraculous recovery, the results of which I had observed downstairs in the physical-therapy room, and heard him say, "Well, if the therapist told you that you would remain paralyzed, you will be. She's had more experience than most of us and you will have to reconcile yourself to this handicap." Then he looked at my heavy, black, flat shoes and the brace attached to it, and smiled again, remarking that he imagined I must formerly have been an elegant and chic young lady and that this new footwear was probably quite out of style for me. There was little I could answer to this left-handed compliment except to ask him to unhinge the knee joint of my long brace so that I could sit down again. But before the neurologist had found the key to the hinge, my husband came forward and mobilized the joint. From then on it became a matter of wry amusement to both of us that every time I wanted to stand up or sit down I would have to ask him to fasten or unhinge my brace.

Dr. Klein, who had watched my skillful husband with some admiration, now said in an encouraging tone: "I have good news for you—we made our definitive diagnosis after the carotid angiogram. You did suffer a CVA and the obstruction is a thrombosis located in the 'bifurcation' of the internal carotid artery." Presumably he meant the internal carotid artery where it divides into the anterior and middle cerebral artery *inside* the skull. Since that was established, he continued, I might as well join society and receive and make telephone calls and receive visitors. Although I never understood the reason for the prohibition against visitors and telephone calls, I somewhat exaggerated my expressions of gratitude and delight about my impending return to my social world.

Hospital Visitors, Flowers, and Futile Comfort

Strangely, it was as though my friends and acquaintances had known about the lifting of the ban that kept me in solitude, except for the constant presence of my husband. For suddenly no more flowers arrived from florists but were hand-delivered, as though my friends had received a secret signal. Those who arrived first were physicians who reacted sensibly to my changed condition. Their principal intent was to comfort me. Oddly enough, most of them claimed to have other friends who had suffered hemiplegia, or even paraplegia, and they told me about the remarkable feats of skill these patients had been able to perform and of their endurance in spite of severe handicaps.

One of these visitors spoke of a friend, an orchestra conductor, of such unique fortitude that *mirabile dictu*, when struck by a CVA his self-control and energy had been such that after a suitable period of convalescence he was able to resume conducting (with one hand, of course). Naturally, all my friends, physicians and others, knew of hemiplegics who had resumed driving their cars after a minimal amount of necessary alterations had been made in their vehicles. And they generally said, "Since you can still use your right hand and foot, actually little has to be done to a car so you can drive it."

Despite their theoretical judgments of my future ability to drive a car, I was never able to do so. I simply did not feel up to coping with the complications of traffic. A possible encounter with a highway policeman would surely have evoked that stream of tears, disabling me and leaving me defenseless.

Not only my medical visitors but also nonmedical ones, who came soon afterwards, remarked on the fact that I looked so well with my pink cheeks. They were all correct: Since early childhood I have had red cheeks; and I assume that this is a peculiar good fortune of a European up-bringing where daily strolls in the fresh air are a must. In fact, when I first came to this country and joined the very sociable circle of Baltimore's suburban citizenry, I was taken aside and advised by a couple of well-meaning matrons that perhaps I should be using a little less rouge. Like my hospital visitors in 1964, the good Baltimore ladies were so unbelieving about the nature of my lively coloring that they wetted their fingertips or used a corner of their handkerchiefs to wipe over my cheek to check the genuineness of my coloring.

By assuring me that I looked so well, my hospital visitors generally felt that they had done enough to comfort me. When I pointed to my totally paralyzed and useless arm and hand, they were apt to repeat over and over again, "But you are fortunate that it is only the left arm and that you still can use your right hand." Since none of them, including the physicians, had experienced even one day of life with a paralyzed extremity, they were incapable of knowing what it was like. Very soon I tired of the repeated irritations caused by these insensitive and uninformed remarks. Well-meant though they were, I had to cut down on the length of their visits by referring to my recurring spells of fatigue. This again often elicited remarks such as: "That's to be expected so soon after a stroke; it'll be much better when you're home or after you've been swimming in a pool." This last addition was derived from the general knowledge that President Roosevelt, by swimming in the pools of Warm Springs, Georgia, had derived much relief from the pain and impediments caused by his attack of poliomyelitis.

Gadgets for Recovery

Actually I had become quite impatient to realize my dream of a visit to a swimming pool. My stay at the hospital, though not excessively long, was fairly uneventful as far as my impediments were concerned. I had become accustomed to my long brace and the ugly, heavy, black, flat-soled shoes to which the brace was attached. But while I was taking my daily walks along the hospital corridor or spending most of my time in bed, odd changes were taking place in my paralyzed extremities.

Owing to my well-trained musculature the contractures, which generally occur after a stroke, became exceptionally strong and my limbs developed a painful rigidity. To prevent what was happening to my left hand, the nurses had given me a fairly large, egg-shaped, gauze ball which I was to hold in my hand at all times to keep my fingers from contracting too tightly. This proved to be quite ineffective as my fingers clenched more and more tightly, so much in fact that eventually my nails lacerated the palm of my hand. Also customary but futile was the pillow inserted into my armpit in order to maintain at least some passive mobility of my rigidly paralyzed shoulder joint and to keep the arm away from my chest. Like the gauze ball the pillow failed to serve its purpose for my shoulder joint remained entirely immobile and developed into a state generally referred to as a "frozen shoulder."

As was to be expected, my left foot underwent contractions similar to my hand; my foot was pulled downward, even though the brace positioned it in its normal state, and I developed what is known as a "drop foot": owing to the foreshortening of the left Achilles tendon, my foot and toes were rigidly pointed down, somewhat like the feet of a ballet dancer on point. The contracture of my left foot gradually became so pronounced that I found it impossible even to think of walking without a brace. I could walk only on the outer edge of my foot and had developed a deformity that looked very nearly like a congenital clubfoot, a talipes varus.

Since all these contractures were very painful, I could no longer rely on the rosy cheerfulness of my complexion to impress my hospital visitors with my bravery. Moreover, I was gradually realizing how devastating my stroke had been and how thoroughly it was to change my life. As a result my visitors, who had come to cheer me up, felt disappointed and let down by what they called my "negative attitude." They nevertheless felt impelled to tell me that I would soon recover completely and surely be able to use my paralyzed arm. Since I had been told repeatedly—and by expert neurologists, physiotherapists, and physiatrists—that there was no such chance after so long a period of rigid paralysis, I could not hide my irritation at the opinionated self-assurance of these lay visitors who "knew" better. Worse still were those who quickly went through the routine of telling me how well I looked and then switched over to a new aspect of consolation: "Be happy it is only one arm: it could have been worse." "How could it have been worse?" was my immediate reply. The ill-humor of my answer left my well-meaning visitors incapable of replying. As was to be expected, such evident lack of serenity served to discourage repeat visits from those I treated so rudely.

Their absence was of some slight advantage for me: I was

able to resume my work on a book that had been half-finished at the time my illness struck. I asked my husband to bring the manuscript from my desk at home as well as the reference books with which I had been working. He did this with much pleasure as he interpreted my will to resume work as a sign of physical as well as emotional recovery. On the following day he transformed my hospital room into a sort of study, far from comfortable but at least making some work possible. Ever more did I become aware of the need for heavy paperweights.

My husband also brought one of our small radios from home, because he knew how much I liked to listen to concert music on the FM stations. This, indeed, gave me much pleasure, but I was faced with an odd incapacity: I was suddenly no longer able to recognize the composer or at least the period of almost any piece that was played. I had less trouble with baroque composers, but certain favorite passages of Brahms, Cesar Franck, and even Beethoven, while seeming familiar, had lost their identity for me, so that I generally had to wait until the announcer informed me of what had just been played. During one of the now infrequent visits by Dr. Klein I told him about this suddenly dimmed ability to recognize selections of classical music. To my surprise he did not seem interested. He merely shrugged his shoulders in a gesture that meant it didn't really matter. Only much later, when I had begun to read up on strokes in the many neurological books I had ordered from the library did I realize that this loss was a frequent concomitant of left-handed strokes. The books similarly explained my inability to make a mental picture for myself of the distances and directions of automobile routes that I had driven innumerable times. They also confirmed my impression that I was apt to lose track of time, and I have often missed an hour or even a day in my reckoning.

To my great and repeated pleasure, my recognition of

music has returned gradually and I am again able to distinguish Brahms from Beethoven, Cesar Franck from Schubert, just to name a few, and to experience many hours of great joy listening to music. I am, however, still entirely incapable of carrying a tune by singing—not even a well-known Christmas carol. While I can make myself hear the melody in my mind, I simply cannot vocalize it.

In my efforts to recapture my music appreciation, Dr. Klein made a suggestion one day that to him must have seemed very helpful. Because he felt I had recaptured full control over my facial muscles, he suggested that I "resume" whistling. This happened to be a friendly suggestion, well-meant, but totally useless for me as I had never whistled before my stroke and have, furthermore, always found whistling an offensive noise, totally unrelated to music.

In other fields I have neither acquired nor regained any special proficiency. Thus, my ability to do simple arithmetic, which never had been entirely satisfactory, has deteriorated somewhat so that I have had to stop keeping my checkbook up-to-date because it would take too long to do the necessary addition and subtraction. Even a calculator is of no help because I could not learn to use it.

In this category of neurologically caused changes belongs an aggravated sensory impairment of my left hand. This includes not only a finger agnosia (i.e., a lack of sensory ability to recognize objects with my left hand) as well as a loss in my ability to recognize the spot that is being touched on the left hand by the examining physician, but also a total lack of recognition of numbers when they are being traced on the palm of my left hand.

From the infrequent visits of the neurologist I gathered that there was really little he or anyone else could do for me; similarly, the daily physical therapy sessions had become repetitious without yielding any new movements or skills. Since I knew that arrangements could be made at home for further physiotherapy and visits of a neurologist if such became necessary, and since I realized that a further stay at the hospital would be of little benefit, I quickly decided to conclude my hospital stay forthwith and to return home on the following day. That day, a Sunday, my husband arrived early, and, together with the nurse, helped me put on the same suit I had worn on the ambulance ride to the hospital some five weeks before. Unlike that earlier ride, I now had to wear my heavy, flat, black shoes and the heavy full-length metal brace which I had not yet become adept in folding and unfolding at the knee.

5

Return Home

Following hospital custom, I was placed in a wheelchair and wheeled to the hospital entrance. As was to be expected, my tears began to flow when I saw our car there. To be placed into the front seat was a fairly complicated procedure because of my long, stiff brace. I sobbed throughout our homeward drive with increased recognition of all the familiar streets and landmarks. Eventually, when we entered our suburban village, my husband advised me to pull myself together and stop crying because some acquaintances might happen to see us and accuse him of bringing me home forcibly. Indeed, his sternness proved effective and I was able to stop. It was a lovely, sunny, Sunday morning. I began again to think of the beneficial exercises I could take in our garden and in our friends' swimming pool and became more hopeful in my outlook.

Having always been an ardent swimmer, starting from my childhood on the banks of the Rhine, I was inclined to agree with those who predicted a healing effect from underwater exercise. I could barely wait for my first swim. The soil of our property happened not to be suited for building and maintaining a swimming pool; hence I had to cast about among our friends who owned one, and would let me use it.

My first swim took place jointly with my husband about two months after my return from the hospital and energetic physical therapy. Just to be in the pool was pure joy; the attempt to swim, however, a shattering disappointment. I had assumed, like everyone else, that there was an intrinsic connection between the immersion in warm water and the ability to swim. There is, perhaps, a certain justification for this assumption if the paralysis affects the same two extremities so that the patient has another set of two limbs left that he can use in swimming. It has always been said that President Roosevelt, both of whose legs were paralyzed, had developed an extremely strong and muscular shoulder girdle as well as powerful arms. But having only one arm and one leg, I found myself incapable of keeping my balance, even if I only tried to walk in the shallow end of the pool. It became evident to me immediately upon immersion that I had no chance of keeping afloat, let alone swimming.

Unfortunately our friends who owned the pool were unaware of the total failure of my swimming effort and my utter frustration. Reclining in chairs alongside the pool, they saw me move about in the water and in their great kindness assumed I was having a splendid time of underwater exercise. Eventually my husband said, "We can't go on like this. Either I'll have to carry you about in the water or you'll hold onto my right shoulder with your right arm and try to kick with your legs. Or we'll give up and come out of the pool and drive home." It is difficult to describe my relief at his insight into the futility of my struggle and I decided then and there to end my swimming career. The failure of the swimming expedition was not the only one after my return from the hospital. Over and over again I had to learn, to realize how totally different life would be for me from what it had been before. First of all, I could not drive a car but always had to wait for my husband, friends, and acquaintances to be free to drive me wherever I had to or wanted to go.

As to the former, a daily excursion took me to the physiotherapist, a very capable man to whom I owe much of my present mobility as well as all the techniques of precaution-taking that so far have protected me from falls and from sustaining possible fractures. I began my treatments with him a few days after my return from the hospital. There I had given little thought to my outer appearance, apart from combing my hair every morning and putting on a dab of lipstick from time to time. Somehow, it had not occurred to me that my hair looked somewhat neglected and drab from the many weeks of bedrest, even though the nurses had one day volunteered to take on the enormous trouble of washing and setting my hair. The improvement was temporary, at best, and by the time I began treatment with the local physiotherapist I must have looked so disheveled and neglected that my husband asked him whether he knew of a hairdresser in this neighborhood—which was new to us—who might restore my hair to its former curls and gloss. The therapist nodded and left his little gymnasium for a business that was adjacent to his own. A few minutes later he came back with a wiry-looking, middle-aged man whom he introduced as "Robert the Coiffeur." Robert happened to have a free hour immediately after my treatment and was willing to take me on as a client. He proved to be an entertaining, cheerful, and skillful hairdresser who was to look after my hair once a week for the next seventeen years. Earlier in his life Robert had been an actor. His ability to assume the personalities of many people, including his cats and a dog whom he saw in the category of humans, made him an entertaining and amusing person.

Routine of Daily Life

With my regular visits to the physiotherapist and the hairdresser my life assumed a certain degree of normalcy. Still, I needed assistance for the simplest activities such as getting out of the car, carrying my purse, and entering the various establishments. Furthermore, so long as I had to wear my long leg brace I was unable to go to the bathroom without the help of someone who could operate the button of my knee joint which was out of reach of my right hand. On the whole, I was far more helpless than I thought I would be prior to my discharge from the hospital. It also became evident that my husband's promise to be my second hand had placed an enormous burden upon him because he felt that he always had to be near me so as to help me whenever the need arose. Even two weeks after my return from the hospital, when my long brace was exchanged for one that reached only to the knee and I became somewhat more independently mobile, my husband still was reluctant to leave me alone at home, fearing that with my new-won independence I might stumble and fall. This, in fact, happened a frightening couple of times when he had to come to my assistance. He gave up the fishing expeditions to which he had so looked forward when we moved to California. Even when neighbors or friends offered to "sit" with me, he still felt impelled to stay at home and watch over me.

With the short, knee-high brace I had achieved at least a modicum of independence, feeling secure enough to get out of my bed or chair and visit the bathroom without my husband's help. There is only one major dependence in this somewhat delicate need that I have retained even now, when I no longer have to wear a brace: This is in entering public rest rooms, because their doors are generally closed by springs, so tight that in opening them they resist my one-handed pull or pressure and I need the help of someone who can hold the door open for me.

Resumption of Work at the University

Shortly after having graduated to my short leg brace I resumed my work at the university, which consisted of conducting further research for the book I had in progress and the teaching of graduate students, interns, and residents. A few had been waiting for me to return to work, as they had applied for acceptance as graduate students even before my move to California had been completed. In addition, numerous situations arose in which I was asked to lecture at various hospitals, medical centers, and other universities. In my eagerness to resume work at my old rate I accepted each of these invitations without consulting my husband whom I had never previously consulted about my professional life. But when he asked in response to each invitation: "Did you ask whether there is an elevator?" I became somewhat embarrassed. In my zeal to return to my past way of life, it had never occurred to me to ask mundane questions about such matters as the number of stairs or the presence of an elevator. Needless to say, this cavalier neglect on my part necessitated many return telephone calls, sometimes even leading to the cancellation of one or another of the engagements altogether when it turned out that with my limited capabilities I would have been unable to reach the lecture hall on foot or even by wheelchair.

By that time, about five weeks after my stroke and ever since, I had developed a strong aversion to being transported in a wheelchair or, in fact, to anything that pointed to my state as an invalid. Oddly enough, I never minded carrying a cane. In a form of inverse snobbery, I even began to collect canes, preferably those imported from Italy. Why the preference for Italian-made canes? American walking sticks (note the word "stick" versus the more elegant "cane"!) are thick and heavy orthopedic appliances which fill an entire hand, while the imported canes are slender and leave room for the handle of a purse, and even a book or any other small portable item. My resentment against all external appearances of my stroke directed itself to my permanently useless, clenched as well as painful hand, and I began to cast about for the names of renowned hand surgeons who might be able to elongate or transplant the contracted tendons leading from my wrist into my fingers and keeping them rigidly curled.

The idea of such an operation had come to me through my constant perusal of the literature on stroke rehabilitation. After intensive inquiries, a specialist in hand surgery at a neighboring school of medicine was highly recommended to me. An initial appointment established a pleasant rapport with the youthful surgeon. He assured me of his willingness to undertake the release of the contracted tendons in my left hand, but he was emphatic on one point, namely, that I do not place any false hope on regaining mobility in my hand. Of course, I reassured him, although, had I been absolutely honest with him, I would have had to confess that I had never entirely given up hope for a miraculous return of mobility to my hand. As it turned out, the operation was successful insofar as my fingers were somewhat relaxed and no longer so tightly clenched that my nails lacerated the palm of my hand. The relaxation, reinforced by daily stretching exercises, has given me a lessening of pain except when I yawn or sneeze, at which moments my hand again contracts into a painful, rigid ball.

When the cast was removed from my newly operated hand, the hand surgeon, Dr. Hunter, and my husband were present. Tenderly, the surgeon took my hand out of the cotton-lined cast like an ornament out of a jewel box. It was fortunate that he was the one to unveil my hand, because he did this with so much gentleness and satisfaction in his own work that I suddenly found I did not have to weep. Naturally, the miracle had not taken place for my hand was still the immobile deadweight it had been before the operation, except that I found it easier to stretch my fingers with my right hand. Dr. Hunter instructed me to do this at least once a day, so as to activate the newly transplanted tendons and to keep them mobile. He also called my attention to the horizontal scar on my wrist which was lined with black sutures. A few days later he removed those, and the scar, quite red at first, has become so pale with time that it is nearly white. I feel certain, however, that if I ever came to a sudden end in a major accident, mugging, or some such violent attack upon my body, any coroner or observant physician would probably conclude that the scar on my wrist was the result of an accident or attempted suicide.

The neurological literature about paralyzed extremities, especially the arms, abounds in statements that are not universally applicable because they are based upon observations by individual patients. Thus it is often stated that hemiplegic patients lose awareness (proprioception) of their paralyzed arms and cannot tell where the arm is or whether it is exposed to a painful stimulus. A further peculiarity has been described by a distinguished British neurologist: He observed that an actual hatred developed in many patients toward their useless arm and that they revenged themselves against it by giving it a derogatory name. Although I too feel a sort of irrational hatred toward my stricken arm, it has not occurred to me to invent a name for it. Furthermore, I am always aware of its whereabouts because of the pain caused by the pendulous weight of its contracted muscles. To counteract that pain I tried wearing my arm in a cloth sling tied around the back of my neck. But because of the great weight of this rigid extremity and the fact that the cloth chafed the skin of my neck I had to give up the attempt and have had to get used to the pain. Beyond that, I generally suffer from the sensation that the skin on my left hemiplegic side is much colder than the rest of my body. My paralyzed arm feels cold regardless of whether I wear a short- or long-sleeved dress. This sensation of cold is confined to my arm and my left cheek. It does not affect my leg which also has retained its proprioceptive faculty as it has regained considerable mobility.

Following the operation on my hand I was grateful for the slight relaxation of my fingers, although I noticed with some dismay that my fingers have still remained somewhat curled inward and become more tightly curled when I laugh, yawn, or sneeze. At least my fingernails no longer lacerate the palm of my hand and, gradually, I have become used to the relative relaxation of my fingers as I was also resentfully growing accustomed to having one completely useless hand. I have also retained an actual finger agnosia so that I am unable to tell the examining physician which one of my fingers he is touching with his hand.

Oddly, I must admit that my one-handed state never caused me as much surprise as might have been expected. It was as if I had waited for it to happen all my life. As a child, a few years after I had begun to learn to write, I suddenly became obsessed with concern as to what I would do if I lost the use of one hand—my right hand, of course—

and how I would prepare myself to write with my left. From then on I trained my left hand to do everything my right hand was capable of doing. Much later, when I started to enjoy eating Chinese food with chopsticks, I carried through my old custom by learning to use chopsticks with my left hand. When disaster struck and my left hand became paralyzed, I felt a fleeting regret at having wasted all that effort in training that hand to share all the skills of my right hand.

For years I wondered why I should have developed this fear of one-handedness when I was seven or eight years old, and never came to a satisfactory conclusion. Suddenly now, when imagination had become reality, I found the explanation for my childhood fantasies—poliomyelitis! or rather, the memories of it. There were during the early years of my life several recurring epidemics of polio that afflicted and badly crippled a number of my contemporaries. It was then that the view of leg braces became a frequent sight, usually coupled with my assumption that the brace was causing the limping and badly atrophied leg. But I can't remember seeing a single paralyzed hand among the polio victims of my childhood. Hence I must assume that the precognition of my losing the use of one hand was simply based upon an unsupported imagination of what poliomyelitis could do to me. Without being very aware of it, however, I had in my childhood and youth known one adult person whose arm was weakened by some paralysis or injury. She was my mother's sister, a delicate and very elegant woman, some six or seven years older than my mother and much beloved and admired by her. Early in my youth I came to realize that it was considered improper to mention Tante Katharina's weak arm, and even more to speculate about the reasons for its atrophy.

Only much later did I realize that in my mother's family

and in her own mind any illness that was outwardly disfiguring or even noticeable represented an impairment of the family's reputation, perhaps because of the fear that it might be transmitted by inheritance to the next generation. It is possible that I might not have been so aware of the ravages of poliomyelitis in my young contemporaries had my mother not spoken so much about these "poor crippled children" and the sorrow their mothers must bear to see their children growing up disfigured, limping, and with braces on their legs. It was then that I became sensitive to the words "cripple" and "crippled," so that after 1964, when I suffered the stroke and found my leg encased in a brace, I was emphatic in using the words "invalid" and "handicapped" whenever I had to explain my need for special consideration in parking the car or climbing stairs or avoiding escalators. Every time I heard the word cripple I thought of the children of my youth who bravely limped along our neighborhood, dragging their heavy braces and their atrophied legs. Only once did I hear the word cripple applied to me—just when I thought I had made all possible provisions to avoid it.

It was quite some time after I had returned to work. I asked my secretary to drive me to the opening session of the meeting of the American Psychiatric Association. The parking facilities were very crowded and I asked the young woman to drive me to the entrance of the building in which the meeting was to take place. Naturally, the policeman tried to divert us into the stream of parking cars from which I could not possibly have walked to the entrance of the building. I opened the car window on my side and called to the traffic policeman that I was unable to walk that far as I was severely handicapped. My secretary who had a stronger voice and was closer to the policeman leaned out of her window and said loudly: "The woman can't walk: she is a cripple." There I sat with that despised word in my ears, truly much too crippled to walk the distance to the entrance of the building which housed the meeting.

Although I had been told very early and repeatedly not to expect any improvement of my left hand or arm, I simply was incapable of giving up all hope. This false hope was fostered by the physical therapist who told me of several of his patients whom he had helped to regain mobility in their paralyzed extremities. When he became aware of my skepticism, he arranged for these former patients to drop in at his little gymnasium when I was having my treatments. It always happened that I was so positioned on the massage table that I could see these "cured" women drive up in their cars or see them come in the door, carrying shopping bags in their formerly paralyzed arms. Gradually, I began to suspect that the arrival of these ladies at the time of my treatment was not a coincidence but had been carefully arranged by the physical therapist to enforce my belief in his curative skill. Since my arm did not show the slightest indication of improvement and my initial hopelessness was reinforced over and over again. I realized that the physical therapist had cleverly selected such patients as had made spontaneous recoveries to drop in when I was there so that I could see living examples of his skill. Much to his surprise I said to him quite coolly, "All right, I'll give you two weeks to work a miracle on my arm also, and if we don't succeed I'll stop the futile exercise of coming here." With some hemming and hawing he tried to convince me that I needed further physical therapy to strengthen my weak leg.

Convalescence Open-Ended

In all fairness, I had to admit that he was right and that I had benefited greatly from the walking exercises he taught me. In addition, I learned certain skills from him that I use in ordinary life innumerable times every day. The following examples will illustrate this: I learned from him to put on my left shoe with only the use of my one mobile hand by crossing my left leg over my right knee, by which means my left leg is foreshortened and my foot is close enough so that I can bend forward and slip the shoe on with my right hand. Furthermore, he taught me never to sit down on any chair or any seat whatsoever without first feeling the edge of the chair against the back of my legs so that I learned to gauge the height of the seat, to sit down slowly in the right direction, and to avoid the danger of falling. Let me repeat that truly indispensable rule my therapist taught me: never to sit down on any chair, bench, or sofa without previously touching the front rim of the seat with the calves of both legs just below my knees. This precaution, I feel certain, has helped me avoid falling on many occasions when the seat I sought was either higher or farther removed than I had anticipated.

Another one of his important instructions was how best to obtain help and support from others with whom I happen to be walking. The instinctive gesture of a healthy person in response to seeing one severely handicapped is to take hold of the paralyzed arm with the intention of guiding him or her. The truth, however, is that this helpful intention causes instability and that it is only with the nonparalyzed, healthy side that one can derive support from a helper. Since I have learned not to be in the least embarrassed to ask for assistance from friends, students, or even strangers, I have accustomed myself to request almost automatically that they, please, let me take their left arm. As a rule, this causes a momentary hesitation during which my walking partners retract their proffered right hand and gradually extend their left arm for my support.

Because I had been active in a variety of sports all my

past life, I found the occasional hours of active and passive exercises at the therapist's quite insufficient. Moreover, even the short leg brace was irritating, because it was heavy and the upper leather cuff was closed with a buckle directly under my knee and caused sores on my lower leg. In the literature concerning stroke rehabilitation I found frequent references to an operation to correct my dropfoot, which was due to the contraction of the calf muscle and the Achilles tendon. When I mentioned the possibility of this operation to correct the footdrop to my physical therapist and asked him whether any of his other patients had undergone this form of surgery, his reply was somewhat ill humored. He advised me strongly against any further surgical correction of my contractures because, as I had seen myself in the operation on my hand, surgery could do little to improve the function of a paralyzed limb. I realized that his negative advice and ill-humor were not independent of his fear of losing a regular and well-paying patient should repair of my foot turn out to be successful.

Recovery by Surgery

The rehabilitation literature made it appear as though operations on foreshortened Achilles tendons were a routine matter for most orthopedic surgeons. That I was mistaken in this impression I soon found out when I began to consult orthopedic surgeons. Each one of the four or five I visited nodded knowledgeably when I presented my contracted foot. They also wrinkled their brows when I asked whether they wished to perform the operation and even shook their heads. Such repairs of neurologically caused contractures were an orthopedic specialty that had come into less frequent use, they said, since the near disappearance of poliomyelitis. Eventually I was referred to yet another orthopedist who actually was willing to schedule the operation right away. He warned me, however, not to set my expectations too high for dispensing with my leg brace after the operation.

By now I was accustomed to these medical warnings against excessive optimism and I assured the orthopedist I would welcome any improvement, even if it was not a complete cure of the contracture. This was sheer hypocrisy, as my assurance to the hand surgeon had been. I took it for granted that a successful elongation of the contracted Achilles tendon would surely free me of my brace.

The operation was scheduled for and carried out ten days after my first interview with the last orthopedist. I awoke from the anesthesia feeling well and without any pain. My foot and lower leg were in a cast which I was to keep for about three weeks. This period seemed to pass quickly, especially since the cast was constructed so as to make walking possible. I became a frequent visitor to the corridors where I gained the impression that my manner of walking had become nearly normal.

My first appointment at the orthopedist's office was set for a week after the cast and sutures had been removed. Naturally, I made use of my new-found ability to walk without a brace and was very pleased when I saw the reflection of delight and pride on the orthopedist's face. He suggested that I walk along the corridor past the offices of his partners, both of whom had seen me before the operation, for them to share his pride in the success of his surgery. Even right after surgery, while I was still limping and relying on the support of my cane, I gave myself over to the illusion that my stroke was no longer noticeable in the way I walked. Without the brace and after the removal of the cast, I saw my foot straight, with a normal longitudinal arch and long—much too long—as it always had been. Since adolescence, in fact, the length of my feet had been the bane of my existence. Because my feet were much longer and broader than those of my girl friends, I was convinced that I would grow taller than they. I was disappointed in this expectation and only grew to be of medium height (i.e., 5 feet, 4½ inches, which now is no longer considered medium but rather short). As my feet have, of course, remained longer and wider than normal, it is extremely difficult for me to find shoes that fit. My feet are so much larger than my husband's that my shoes are a bit too big for him. For this reason he can try on and buy shoes for me, thus relieving me of a very difficult and generally frustrating chore.

His shoe-purchasing excursions on my behalf have often led to amusing incidents. Owing to my partial paralysis and the contractures of my leg I can walk only on flat-heeled shoes; even a low heel makes me feel insecure. Therefore my husband, on his buying trips for my shoes, has had to go to the women's department in shoe stores or into shoe stores that cater to women only and has had to ask for flat heeled pumps, size 9½ C. Occasionally he has returned triumphant from these buying trips, with one or two pairs that fit him comfortably and hence also were comfortable for me. On other occasions he came home hugely amused about some of his efforts to try on women's shoes that fit him. The condition that these shoes should be flat-heeled usually caused particular difficulties because of their scarcity. In fact, a shoe salesman (never a saleswoman) sometimes would say to him with a sly wink, "But wouldn't *you* rather have some shoes with heels?" My husband rarely took the time to convince the salesperson that he was not a transvestite and was not buying the shoes for himself.

In spite of these occasionally frustrating incidents, my husband's patience and helpfulness never lessened, and for every pair of shoes, that is, for every step I have taken since I suffered my stroke, I am indebted to his persistence in obtaining fitting footwear for me. In doing so he has also facilitated my professional life as a university professor and made it possible for me to give the lectures that are part of my duties. Since he usually drives me to the hospitals or universities where I am to lecture, he always carries a folded wheelchair in the trunk of our car to spare me the strenuous walks on long university corridors. With his constant awareness of my various handicaps he has made it possible in the past twenty years for me to fulfill the demands of my profession and to be at least as productive and creative as I had been in the many years prior to my stroke.

There is one handicap that I don't seem to be able to overcome however: A severe backache that I experience after sitting at my desk for too long. For instead of sitting straight, I feel my left shoulder drooping together with the dead weight of my left arm. My normal right side has to carry its own weight as well as that of my left.

The Specter of Overweight

Naturally, my physicians have always warned me against gaining weight. I find myself deploring this further deprivation of "all the good things in life." Dieting has in fact been a dread throughout the twenty years of my illness. When I was first admitted to the hospital in March 1964, the internist who had been consulted by my neurologist asked me about my weight, I replied honestly that since giving up smoking I had gained at least ten pounds. No sooner had I made it, I regretted the confession, for the internist replied complacently: "Well, then we know the cause of your stroke—it's simply overweight—and we'll combat it by placing you on a 1,200 calorie diet."

Take the desolation that accompanies a stroke, add to it the tastelessness of lukewarm institutional food, top it by a steady sensation of hunger never satisfied by the insufficient quantities of that hospital food. The degradation of hunger pangs was heightened by another measure introduced by the internist. This was the bed scale, a huge instrument, somewhat like an ironing board, at bed level that rested on top of a scale. This machine was wheeled into my room every morning after breakfast, two orderlies lifted me on to it, and my daily weight was noted and inscribed onto a curve. Needless to say, since the weighing took place every day the variations of weight were minimal to say the least, and the curve, rather like a horizontal line, did not begin to descend as long as I was in the hospital.

Even after my discharge from the hospital I began to lose weight only after I developed a severe loss of appetite, aggravated by vomiting spells, whenever I forced myself to eat a full meal. I had always been very slim and had only gained weight after I gave up smoking to "stay healthy." When I realized that the "Surgeon General's Warning" had failed its purpose in my case, I simply decided to resume smoking in a very moderate amount. It seems I have been smoking so moderately that I have scarcely lost any of the weight I had gained when I stopped smoking three years earlier. However, whatever I tried so far as my weight and appetite were concerned, it was evident that I had lost enough weight to walk fairly easily, especially when I watched my posture. It was evident also that I would never regain the pleasure in eating that I had experienced before.

In addition to the depressing time and the daily weighing I had experienced in the hospital, I was burdened by another memory that succeeded in ruining my pleasure in food. That memory was a leftover of my childhood, when my mother, a tall and slender woman, tried her best to achieve a similarly slender disposition in me. There was scarcely a meal at my parents' house when she wouldn't say about one item or another that was served, be it potatoes or dessert, "Ilza, is it really *necessary* for you to eat all that? Don't you want to stay slim?" I knew full well that this admonition was not addressed solely to me, but actually more to my father, whose inclination to plumpness my mother feared I had inherited. There was a silent conspiracy between my father and me to leave my mother's admonitions and rhetorical questions unanswered and to eat as much as we pleased. As a result of my mother's frugal eating habits she would, for instance, never have soup or dessert served to her at dinner. I simply adored those family friends or relatives at whose homes food was hugely enjoyed. As I was usually invited there together with my parents, I remained under my mother's ever-watchful eyes.

My eating style now has been based largely upon keeping myself on a low-calorie diet. So whenever I have to look after my own meals, I eat a hard-boiled egg together with a cup of low-fat yogurt, neither of which requires any difficult preparation. To facilitate our home life my husband, who had taken over the complete household, including the shopping and cooking, fortunately was not ambitious to become a gourmet cook and prepare complicated dishes. Moreover, for the sake of our health he confines himself mostly to broiled meats, tossed salads, and cooked vegetables, such as asparagus and cauliflower. Fortunately for both of us, we like some of the frozen dishes which are tasty, well-seasoned, and easy to serve. In spite of my careful diet I have not been able to avoid gaining weight, which is probably due largely to my almost complete lack of physical exercise. In memory of my humiliating encounters with the bed scale at the hospital, I have now stopped weighing myself, but leave the control over my weight and appearance to the mirror and the waistbands of my skirts as well as the notches of my belts.

Learning to Cope

When it became evident that the profit derived from daily lessons at the physical therapist's was not commensurate with the time and effort involved in my frequent trips to his little gymnasium, my husband and I decided to reduce these visits to twice a week, because it was easy for me to perform his exercises every morning of the remaining days of the week at home. In fact, I found it gratifying to invent new exercises and add them to my program.

In everything I did, and still am doing, I have been particularly concerned to keep my balance so as to protect myself from falling, since I know I would be incapable of getting up by myself and might have to lie on the floor with an injury, or even a fracture, until someone happened to come along and help me get up. At home this worry was not too serious as I was rarely alone and was generally protected by my husband's presence and the soft carpeting on the floor. It was different on the days that I went to the university, where I either had office hours and conferred with students and colleagues or gave lectures and seminars. Because I am incapable of carrying my books or lecture notes, I have had to make arrangements with a secretary or one of the students to carry my teaching materials for me. Not infrequently, it happened that a pen, pencil, or worksheet would fall to the floor. If this happened when anyone was present in my office, the visitor would quickly bend down and pick up the fallen object. Because I was so dependent upon others for nearly all undertakings, I decided to teach myself to bend down and pick up whatever had fallen to the floor. Initially I found this to be a daring undertaking, as I was unable to bend my left knee and felt slightly out of balance. Eventually, however, I learned to bend down so quickly that I had no time to think about loss of balance and just took hold of the fallen object. The awkward aspect of my bending-down-and-picking-up exercises was that since I always have to have my cane in my hand I have to use my index finger and thumb to get hold of the object on the floor. In order to improve my skill in bending down and picking up fallen objects, I took a little box of buttons and emptied it repeatedly upon the floor. After I had bent down ten or twenty times and collected all the buttons, I knew I had improved my skill and steadiness. Because I am restricted to the use of two fingers for holding my cane when picking up fallen objects from the floor, I often must make use of the readily proffered help of others.

My original intention in learning how to pick up fallen objects from the floor was mainly to spare my husband the need to walk unnecessary distances. If, for instance, my cane should fall on the floor, as so often happens, I used to feel helpless without it, but now I can pick it up myself. However, this recently won independence of being able to pick up things from the floor also has its negative aspects: When a stranger or a friend helpfully hurries to my side to pick up a fallen object, my newly acquired reflex makes me bend down and anticipate the helpful gesture. I suppose this is to a large extent the result of the early and often fairly rough training I experienced from physiatrists, physical therapists, and other rehabilitation experts. They absolutely refused to lend me a hand even on occasions that ordinary social politeness would have required their assistance.

As an example, I would like to relate a meeting with a physiatrist of considerable national reputation whom I consulted when I happened to give a guest lecture in the midwestern hospital where he practiced. When I was about to leave his office, I slipped into the left sleeve of my coat with some difficulty and looked at the physiatrist expectantly, waiting for him to hold my coat so that I could slip into my right sleeve. Instead of doing what any well-bred man would do automatically to help a woman into her coat, this specialist in rehabilitative medicine pulled off my coat from the left arm and shoulder where I had been holding it with some precarious balance. He let it fall to the ground and said: "Now pick it up and put it on again; some day later you will be grateful to me for having made you do it." As a result of this shocking form of "education" in independence, I often find myself refusing help in a way that must appear incomprehensibly brusque to those who wish to assist me.

Naturally, there are many occasions during each working day when I need and gratefully accept help from a variety of persons. This help begins with my arrival at the hospital to which I am generally driven by a medical colleague who lives in our neighborhood. Apart from the comfort of having this transportation, I enjoy our weekly conversation and communication of medical and social news. When we arrive at the entrance to the hospital I am usually met by one of the departmental secretaries who comes downstairs to carry my purse and briefcase since I cannot carry both in addition to my cane in my one available hand. Most physical therapists, occupational therapists, and other rehabilitation specialists would interrupt my narrative here to tell me about all sorts of inventions by means of which pocketbooks and briefcases could be attached to long leather straps and hung over my shoulder, so that my hand would not be involved. It is true I have seen advertisements of such shoulder bags and even briefcases and have tried them out, but I found them entirely impractical. The straps simply slip off my shoulder since

I lack the ability to raise my shoulder so as to counterbalance the weight of the bag.

The rehabilitation specialists who practice and teach occupational therapy know an endless number of methods to teach the handicapped to help themselves and to live near-normal daily lives, such as the conversion of a handbag into a shoulderbag. Because most of this occupational therapy is very complicated and time-consuming, I simply tried to ignore it when I first should have been practicing it, right after my stroke. But at that time I was still involved in my efforts to deny my handicap and in thinking of it as transitory. When gradually I became convinced that I would be paralyzed forever and that no earthly or higher power could return my life-style to a normal one, it was too late for me to make up for all the techniques I had not learned; I had become too stiff and awkward.

To my husband's sorrow I have developed a compulsion that must be distressing and tiresome to him and to all my friends. It is a preoccupation with my former appearance, when I appeared tall and slim, my legs appeared long and elegant in high-heeled shoes, and my face had its original lean contours. The change in my face to its present broad shape and excessively round cheeks is the consequence of several cortisone injections that I received a few years after my stroke to lessen the severe pain I was suffering—and still am—in my left sacroiliac region. Even though the cortisone injections were aimed into the bursa of my hip joint, the substance made itself felt systemically and caused the typical facial swelling which has not lessened in all the years since it first became noticeable. My absorption with my former appearance recently received another blow when I saw a new passport picture, hurriedly taken in color, which showed that I do have some slight facial paralysis. Until then the mirror had been able to hide this disfigurement from me and I had deluded myself into believing that I had been spared this unfortunate concomitant of a stroke. My discovery of this disfigurement on the passport photo reminded me of a vignette I had observed more than twenty years earlier in the physical-therapy room of the hospital, when an older woman (probably my age!) was pushed into the room in a wheelchair. The chair came to rest directly in front of a large, wall-size mirror, so that the woman could see herself and take stock of her appearance. The striking feature in her outward aspect was that one half of her face, evidently the hemiplegic side, was contracted so that one eyelid was closed and her mouth appeared half-open. How lucky am I, I thought then, to have been spared this unfortunate blow. I am not quite certain how I had come to the conclusion that I had no facial paralysis: I simply must assume that I never had come face to face with myself unexpectedly in a mirror, but always had had the time to arrange my features in a satisfactory expression.

But now I can no longer delude myself in this matter and simply have to accept the reality of the passport photo and the knowledge that one side of my face is markedly contracted. This also, I now know, accounts for my tendency, first remarked upon by the neurologist, Dr. Klein, to lose bits of food while eating, so that I must never forget to wipe not only my mouth after eating, but also all adjacent areas, including my chin, because things like soups, sauces, and salad dressings are apt to wander about around my mouth. Added to what I consider to be part of a facial paralysis, there is a slight facial hypesthesia, a diminished tactile sensibility that interferes with my ability to feel the results of a runny nose on the hemiplegic side. In both cases my husband calls my attention to the mishap with a gesture or a soft-spoken word. He has also been my unrelenting critic in my lecturing career since I had the stroke.

Initially, I was aware of some shortcomings myself,

such as my inclination to talk too fast and my inability to modulate my voice or to make the appropriate pauses between sentences. I know that I was further handicapped in lecturing by doing so while sitting down rather than standing up, in which position I was better able to project my voice. But standing for nearly an hour, actually supported by only one leg, has proved difficult and painful; hence I have conquered my vanity and learned to lecture sitting down. Control of my voice has benefited greatly from a number of sessions with a speech therapist, who had also worked with several prominent politicians, and I was able to renew my self-confidence even when I spoke in a sitting position. The most regrettable change in my career as a lecturer occurred in my new inability to speak without a manuscript. Gone are the days when I spoke freely with only a few notes before me. Now I am afraid either of condensing my subject into too brief a summary of the lecture I prepared or conversely—and adversely—of being too long-winded without the limits and limitations of a manuscript. Furthermore, I frequently lecture in foreign languages and cannot be absolutely certain that the essential vocabulary is available to me just when I need it.

Pain and Acupuncture Therapy

Like anyone else I am frequently asked, "How are you?" to which I have learned to reply without any hesitation, "Fine, thanks." No one, I know, wants to know that I am far from "fine," that I am miserable to be a permanent invalid. Indeed the factual answer would be: "I am as well as I'll ever be." Unfortunately, contrary to the expectations of most laymen, being partially paralyzed is a painful affliction. The contracture of my leg causes a tilt of my pelvic girdle and with it a curve in my vertebral column. No analgesic helps this permanent pain for any length of time; hence I have tried whatever other orthodox and unorthodox treatments were available. I have been hypnotized, and tried self-hypnosis; I have tried biofeedback, gradual and total relaxation, and found none to be of any avail. As was to be expected, the neurologists washed their hands of me because my pain did not actually have a neurological cause. So I tried what in my case was the logical last recourse—acupuncture. I say it was the logical recourse for me, as I had written and published articles, books, and material about acupuncture decades before most Westerners knew how to spell the word. In fact, the first article on acupuncture published in the *Journal of the American Medical Association* was written by me in May 1962 upon the invitation of the editor who had long known of my preoccupation with the study of this ancient and exotic treatment.

Now that all other Western means of alleviating pain had failed, I turned to acupuncture and was fortunate in finding it helpful for certain lengths of time. Initially, I was free of pain after acupuncture treatments for two to three days; gradually the intervals could be extended to a week and, eventually, even to two weeks before the pain returned acutely and was stilled with another treatment. In the choice of my acupuncture therapist I have been exceptionally fortunate. Born and raised in China, she had received a broad classical education there and, subsequently, a Western scientific education in the United States. She had studied acupuncture as a young girl and kept abreast of new developments in China by following the scientific literature on the subject. Together with her and with her husband who is an American-trained surgeon, I rounded out my own studies on acupuncture by writing a textbook on the subject that is based entirely on current Chinese publications.* It has proved to be so successful that the first edition was sold out in less than a year and we had to prepare a second edition soon after.

Fortunately, my acupuncturist also uses moxa heating of the needles, a time-honored Chinese practice which greatly increases the efficacy of simple acupuncture. Moxa is a word derived from the Japanese *mogusa* (burning herb), and consists of the leaves of dried wormwood (i.e., artemisia moxa), which are crumbled into fine grains or dust and combined in a big roll. When lighted, this moxa roll burns slowly, emitting strong heat and an incenselike scent. The burning moxa roll is held some three-fingers' breadth away from the acupuncture needle and its point of insertion into the skin. The odor of the glowing wormwood and its sensation of heat upon the skin have a wonderfully soothing effect which alleviates the pain, not only instantly but also for a protracted period of time.

The attacks of migraine and simple headaches from which I had been suffering on and off before my stroke have practically ceased since the CVA, with the exception of the episodes of scintillating scotoma, which come on from time to time and are very frightening and disturbing to me. Since such scotomas were the forerunners of my stroke, I am deeply concerned each time I suffer one now that it might be a harbinger of another stroke. But as they generally do not last much longer than twenty-five to thirty minutes, I have so far convinced myself that they are due to transitory vascular spasms and therefore may not represent a further lasting threat to my health.

It may appear odd and incongruous that I can now,

---

*Leong T. Tan, Margaret Y. C. Tan, and Ilza Veith. *Acupuncture Therapy: Current Chinese Practice*. Philadelphia: Temple University Press, 1976.

partially paralyzed as I am, actually speak of my present condition as "my state of *health*" and hope it will persist in its current state to which I have become accustomed. Fortunately, I have been advised to take a daily dose of Inderal (propranolol) and have experienced far fewer scotomas since I have been on this medication.

On the other hand, I have not lost all anxiety that I might suffer another stroke the next time in the left side of my brain, which would deprive me of the use of my right hand and, worse still, even of my ability to speak. Of course I am also aware that I might have another stroke in the right side of my brain and that my present handicaps, which I have overcome in part, may become aggravated. In contrast to former times I regularly see my internist and have my blood pressure taken. For a brief time he found it to be elevated, but soon succeeded in controlling it by means of appropriate medication.

There is considerable doubt as to the cause of my stroke; there have been few cases where a migraine attack has resulted in a permanent occlusion and destruction because of lack of oxygen that is normally carried by the blood. I seem to be one of these rare cases. Other such cases were described by the great neurologist, Jean-Martin Charcot, in his extraordinarily interesting chapter "Scintillating Scotoma," from his *Clinical Lectures on Diseases of the Nervous System* (pp. 63–68, which was published in London in 1889 and delivered in the Infirmerie of the Salpètrière in Paris in 1889).

It is difficult to think of anyone but a neurologist of Charcot's intellectual dimensions as being able to describe a phantom vision such as scintillating scotoma as realistically as he did. First, it seems as graphic as the illustration in the chapter on "Scintillating Scotoma" that he renamed "ophthalmic migraine." Charcot spoke of it in the following way:

CLINICAL LECTURES

ON

DISEASES OF THE NERVOUS SYSTEM

DELIVERED AT

THE INFIRMARY OF LA SALPÊTRIÈRE

BY

PROFESSOR J. M. CHARCOT,

PROFESSOR IN THE FACULTY OF MEDICINE OF PARIS; PHYSICIAN TO THE SALPÊTRIÈRE; MEMBER OF THE INSTITUTE, AND OF THE ACADEMY OF MEDICINE OF FRANCE; PRESIDENT OF THE SOCIÉTÉ ANATOMIQUE, ETC.

VOLUME III
(CONTAINING EIGHTY-SIX WOODCUTS).

TRANSLATED BY

THOMAS SAVILL, M.D.Lond., M.R.C.P.L.,

MEDICAL SUPERINTENDENT OF THE PADDINGTON INFIRMARY, LONDON; HONORARY MEMBER OF THE SOCIÉTÉ ANATOMIQUE, PARIS; FORMERLY ASSISTANT PHYSICIAN AND PATHOLOGIST TO THE WEST LONDON HOSPITAL.

LONDON:
THE NEW SYDENHAM SOCIETY.

1889.

Fig. 1. Title page

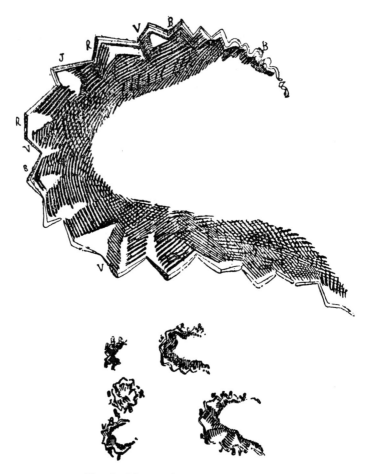

Fig. 2. Phases of Scintillating Scotoma

The Return Home

"I will simply remind you that in an ordinary attack of ophthalmic migraine of the typical kind, a luminous figure appears in the visual field, which is at first circular, then semicircular, of a zigzag shape like the drawing of a fortification. Agitated with a very rapid vibratory movement, the image is sometimes white and phosphorescent. . . . The scotoma is often replaced by a temporary hemianopsia of the field of vision so that the patient sees only half the object. . . . Vomiting terminates the attack and the patient gets well again."

This brief description of the average case of ophthalmic migraine is followed by the case history of a young man who had five attacks in rapid sequence which deprived him of his ability to speak and movement of the right half of his body.

6

Dreams: Hopeful and Threatening

For a long time, it seems, I had not accepted my hemiplegic state as a fact of life and as a permanent fate. This became evident from the content of my dreams in which I invariably saw myself in my prestroke surroundings, without paralysis or any handicap whatever. In my dreams I also had my parents with me and many of those friends and relatives who are no longer part of my present life. Naturally, I cherished those dreams in which I saw myself in good health and in full command of all my faculties and extremities. Immediately on awakening, I usually made brief notes of the dream contents in order to be able to reconstruct the dream in the course of the day. Eventually I tired of the futility of deluding myself with snatches of my hopeful imaginings and stopped making notes of my dreams. Shortly afterward, in fact, realism began to take over my dream life and I have since seen myself as helpless and handicapped in my dreams, as I actually am. To make matters worse, in my dreams I have transferred my own severe handicap onto my husband, who is the mainstay of my existence.

In the first such terrible dream I placed us both in a new restaurant that was built on various levels, connected with one another with short but steep stairs. In my dream I was following him from one room into the other and was waiting for him to turn back and take my arm when I saw him falter and collapse, until finally two waiters noticed the mishap and carried him away in a different direction from where I was standing. This was the end of that dream and left me helpless and desperate. Other dreams, equally frightening, have also placed me in distressing situations from which I found myself unable to escape, because of my own incurable handicap. After seventeen years of self-deception in my dreams, the last year presented to me a reality so shocking and disabling that I was incapable of escaping from the threatening situation in which my dreams had placed me. Again my dreams became so violent that I screamed in self-defense until I was shaken awake by my husband. After some nights that were filled with frightening dreams, I often found myself blinded by scintillating scotoma at breakfast and deeply afraid of their portent.

Dreams, good and bad, have influenced my moods and well-being in the past twenty years. Here, I should emphasize that I have always dreamed a great deal, and so vividly that the dream content has usually remained with me throughout the following day. There is, in fact, a certain dream that I dreamed more than fifty-five years ago, when I still lived in Germany, that dealt with life in the United States before I had even set foot on its shores. It is that dream I still remember vividly. The same is also true of most of the dreams I have had since I have been an invalid.

In talking about dreams and sleep, I must refer again to my early weeks in the hospital immediately after I had experienced my CVA, when Dr. Klein declined to give me any sleeping medication for fear that it might obscure my symptoms and hence also the diagnostic and etiological aspects of my illness. As a consequence I slept poorly during the night, perhaps because I took frequent naps for short periods during the daytime. But at night, when the hospital went to sleep, the lights were turned out, and the corridors fell silent, I continued to read until my eyes were so fatigued that they became unable to focus on the print. When finally I fell asleep, probably between eleven and twelve o'clock at night, I generally woke again between two and four o'clock in the morning and remained awake until five o'clock, beset by anxiety about my future life as an invalid and my fears about a possible premature end to my beloved academic career.

When I was discharged from the hospital and again slept in my own bed at home, the diagnosis of the location and nature of my stroke had been made and there was nothing that could still be obscured by sleeping pills. Therefore I decided that my sleepless nights and tormented wakeful hours early in the morning could no longer serve any reasonable diagnostic purpose and I helped myself to the sleeping pills that I had left over from the time before my stroke. Immediately, I began to spend the nights in long, deep, and restful sleep, enjoying dreams about my healthy past when I was slim and mobile enough to play tennis and swim in the ocean or any pool or lake.

After my supply of sleeping pills had been exhausted I tried to return to sleep without medication. Again it took several hours of tossing and turning in bed and of arduous concentrated thought of my current and future research projects before I fell into a short and restless sleep. The wakeful hours between 2 A.M. and 4 A.M. again exhausted me with gloom, until I achieved my last hour of early-morning sleep.

When I was finally able to replenish my supply of sleeping pills, I returned to many hours of restful sleep. In the vast literature of the various sleep researchers I had always noted their emphasis on the beneficial effect of dreaming and its absolute necessity for the maintenance of good mental health. It was also believed by these sleep researchers that drug-induced sleep interfered with dreaming, probably because they could observe very little REM (Rapid Eye Movement) sleep in the various "sleep laboratories" after the patients had been given sleeping medication.

In contrast to the scientists' research findings, I observed that in my case at least (an entirely insufficient "sample of one"), medication does not interfere with my dreaming and that my dreams continue to be as lively and memorable as ever before. Whether they are accompanied by Rapid Eye Movement, I am, of course, unable to say. So as not to become completely habituated to the taking of sleeping pills, I decided to take one every second night and, later, every third night. In doing so I evolved a fairly satisfactory sleeping pattern for myself. Depending on the time I go to bed and stop reading, I fall asleep fairly promptly even when I have not taken a sleeping drug. But when I sleep without medication, I always have to suffer through two or three hours of early-morning wakefulness. This pattern of interrupted sleep has persisted throughout the past twenty years, and I have allowed myself a rhythm of sleep medication every two or three nights, alternating with drug-free sleep.

Another serious interference with restful sleep is the contracture and rigidity of my left paralyzed extremities. My "frozen shoulder," which has never fully relaxed, often develops painful cramps at night, together with my elbow joint, which I cannot extend for more than a minute without strenuous efforts of assistance from my healthy arm. Early in my rehabilitation career one of the many physiatrists I consulted suggested that I take ten milligrams of Valium three times a day in order to loosen my contracted arm. While at that time this regimen did little to relax my muscles, I discovered that a single Valium tablet of five milligrams at night helps a bit in relaxing my cramped muscles and also allows me to go back to sleep.

While the problem of dressing, undressing, or changing my clothes had been comfortably solved at home with the endless patience of my husband—who has learned to struggle with zippers, buttons, and folds of material—I have not, in the twenty years of my paralysis, developed the skill to open or close my zipper closings in the front or back of my dresses, or in dressing myself. From my ability to put on knit cardigans and other light jackets without help, I rather feel that I have not developed any apraxia in dressing. The one reason I cannot dress without help is the paralysis of my left hand. For I am told that patients with left-sided hemiplegia may lose the ability of associating the structure of their clothes with the appropriate parts of their bodies. Perhaps I could develop a greater skill and independence if I disposed of all my clothes and purchased others that are wide and loose and button in front. If they also had elastic closing of the sleeves I would be able to dress myself as, even now, I can put on my brassiere by fastening its hooks and eyes before stepping into the garment and pulling it up over my body so that I can slip into its elastic shoulder straps. The variety of changes I could contemplate to facilitate my dressing are endless and, equally endless, are the numbers of skills I should teach myself to make up for my one-handed state.

There are, of course, many occasions when my helplessness in dressing or seating myself becomes evident to strangers. It is on occasions such as when I am about to put on or take off a sweater in a restaurant that a total stranger will hurry over from his or her table with the sincere intention of being helpful and try to force whichever one of my arms is nearest to him or her into the sleeve of my cardigan without knowing that I must follow a precise sequence of movements in putting on or taking off garments. This sequence of movements in dressing and undressing is part of the early curriculum of occupational therapy; it decrees that in dressing as a hemiplegic person, one must first slip on the sleeve of one's paralyzed arm and, in undressing, one has to slip off the sleeve of one's healthy arm first.

If, as so often happens in restaurants, a helpful soul hurries over from another table and tries to assist me in pulling on a sweater, coat, or whatever other garment, feeling I am in need of their help, they often cannot be discouraged even by a forceful rejection. There have been numerous other occasions when strangers have felt called upon to prove their helpful intentions without the slightest thought that it takes a certain amount of skill and technique to assist a partially paralyzed person, and that it might be a more sensible approach to preface one's proffered help by inquiring, "How can I help you?" In numerous such cases when I have had to discourage uninvited and unskilled assistance, the person who has rendered it appears deeply hurt and annoyed by my "ingratitude."

Another frequent reaction on the part of strangers who pass me, especially when I am carried along in a wheelchair, is that they smile at me in what they assume to be a compassionate manner. Although I usually derive little comfort from this strange token of compassion, I have learned to force myself to return the uninvited smile. Similarly, I have taught myself to give a noncommittal reply when strangers ask me whether I have suffered an accident or whether something else has happened to me.

In the European hotel where we usually spend our summer holidays, we tend to meet the same people year after year. They are quite observant and obviously curious about the minor alterations in my manner of walking. Although it has not really changed much in the past seven years since we've been going to this particular resort. I am told by friends and strangers alike that I am now walking so much better. Naturally, I express my appreciation for their concern and interest. In this year, my appearance must have been a letdown to my well-wishers because I was in a wheelchair that was being pushed by my indefatigable husband. My relegation to the wheelchair is due to very severe pains in my left knee which become aggravated whenever I walk long distances. Since the x-rays did not reveal any arthritic changes in the knee joint and I had noticed that extended rest ameliorated the pain, my husband not only volunteered but insisted on my traveling the long distances of the hotel in the wheelchair that accompanies us on all our travels.

This wheelchair is a particularly practical model for our purposes as it is light and can be folded easily to fit into the trunk of almost any car. Having our own wheelchair along relieves us of dependence upon wheelchairs of hotels and airports, although the latter's vast distances necessitate our requesting the help of porters or airline employees who know their way through the immense installations and the hidden locations of the elevators, as I am incapable of using escalators. Nevertheless, our overseas travels are very difficult for my husband, who has to find porters for our large, cumbersome suitcases, hand luggage, and the wheelchair as well as locate customs and immigration; all this requires repeated negotiations with the airlines in order to receive their promised assistance.

If it sounds strange that every year my husband, in his advanced eighties, would undertake these strenuous trips to Europe, the Far East, or the South Pacific, it can be explained only by the fact of the endless kindness and compassion with which he attempts to open the doors of my prison of paralysis and to compensate for my inability to participate in the social and cultural activities of my friends and colleagues. In addition to my joy in visiting foreign friends and countries, these trips also fulfill an important professional purpose in that they make it possible for me to continue my professional contact with foreign colleagues. In fact, whenever I make it known in Germany, New Zealand, or Japan that I will be visiting these countries in the near future, I generally receive invitations to give guest lectures on whatever subject I happen to be currently carrying on research. Thus, apart from giving me the joy of traveling, these annual trips enable me to maintain professional contacts throughout the world and encourage me to engage in continued research.

While I am always aware of the precarious state of my health and the possibility of suffering additional disabling disease, I have been able to keep this fear under some control, in contrast to another fear that rarely ever leaves my mind. It is the fear that some unfortunate accident or illness might befall my husband and, apart from the joy of his company and his understanding of my needs, I would be left alone and totally helpless.

To make up for the time, the equanimity, and the variety of services he renders me, I would have to engage a number of helpers, including a driver and even a nurse to help me take a bath. All these services would have to be prearranged according to a fixed schedule as I am entirely incapable of leaving our house by myself, because it is built on a hill. The driveway is so steep that I can neither walk down to the street nor climb back up into the house. Even such mundane thoughts as my having to shop or go to the bank by myself and look after my economic needs are incredibly frightening. I don't know how I would be able to get to the bank and up the few steps by myself, not to speak of carrying a purse or a briefcase with the necessary papers. A further impossibility would be my opening one of the heavy wooden doors that lead inside. I am so possessed by the fear that something might happen to my husband that I worry about him incessantly when we are not together.

From the suddenness of my own cerebral vascular accident, I know how quickly and unexpectedly such total incapacity can befall anyone, so that I am in fear of it for my husband whenever an unexpected delay keeps him from me when he is away from home for any reason. If he is marketing while I am waiting for him in the parked car outside the store and I become aware of an uncommon delay in his return, I generally wonder how I might be able to get out of the car and close all its doors and lock them, so that I could follow him into the store to discover what might have happened to him. So far he has always returned just when I had mapped out the logistics of my search expedition, and these thoughts have made me feel silly about my exaggerated anxiety.

7
Afterthoughts

It is largely my dreams that make me aware of the intensity of my anxious preoccupation with my husband's health and his ability to continue functioning as "my second hand." The most frightening of my recent dreams was probably inspired by the many reports we heard in Germany, and all over Europe, of burglaries and muggings in that formerly highly law-abiding country. So insecure have German citizens become about their security and the safety of their belongings that they have evolved complicated alarm and security systems whenever they are away from home, be it for a vacation, a single evening, or just part of a day.

Even though burglaries and muggings are just as frequent in our country and neighborhood, my husband shrugs off this possibility, fully convinced that were he ever to be confronted by invaders or burglars in our home, the former reflexes of his youthful boxing training would be set in motion and he would be able to cope easily with intruders physically, regardless of his being an octogenarian. Almost as unrealistic as my husband's theories about his ability to defend himself and me physically are my preparations for my one-handed defense against a violent intruder. My canes, one of which is always in reach of my right hand, could serve as excellent weapons of defense. Two of these canes are lined with steel rods and are therefore nearly unbreakable. The golden handle of my gold-headed cane is heavy and has sharp edges. Apart from the fantasies of physical self-defense in my home, I have made preparations to call for help without being noticed by an intruder. Next to the chair in which I spend most of my days when I am at home, I have a small "slim-line" telephone with touch buttons. In preparation for unexpected events, such as electric-light failures, I have trained myself to find the numbers of the local police and fire departments in the dark with the thumb of my right hand.

Owing to the spasticity of my left hip joint and leg, I am often overcome at night with severe pain in my sciatic nerve. So severe indeed is this pain that I feel a burning sensation in the entire course of the nerve, from its beginning in the gluteal muscle down to my heel. That additional problem was diagnosed when I consulted neurologists at the Mayo Clinic about four years after the onset of the CVA, while I was there as a visiting lecturer. My sciatica is no doubt a complication of the hemiplegia, owing to the tilting of my pelvis and the herniation of my fifth lumbar disc. In addition to Valium, I have found that I can relieve the sciatic pain by elevating my knees with a pillow I always keep next to my bed so that I can pull it up and place it under my knees whenever it becomes necessary. Besides, I still experience marked relief from the nightly attacks of pain thanks to getting periodic acupuncture treatment. Usually the relief lasts for two to three weeks; afterwards the sciatic pain returns not only at night but also in the daytime, especially when I sit at my desk for any length of time.

In spite of the see sawing of pain and well-being that has gone on for more than twenty years, together with the unrelieved handicap of hemiplegia, I have been able to continue my professional life with hardly any hindrance and with the same satisfaction in my achievements that I might have felt had I been in perfect health. Apart from many publications, a great joy in my academic career has been my warm relationships with colleagues and students, relationships that have often turned into affectionate friendships, continuing in several cases for decades.

My secret and unrealistic wish of complete recovery from the paralysis has gradually gone the way of all dreams in having disappeared from my consciousness. Still present, however, is the depression that often accompanies strokes as the result of the devastation of my former life. With considerable effort and self-control I have generally succeeded in presenting a cheerful facade not only on social and public occasions but even to myself.

At times my feelings of depression become overwhelming, and I consider returning to a psychiatrist. However, after a few tentative conversations with psychotherapists I have felt neither comforted nor relieved of my depression. Nor was I convinced that this method would have any therapeutic value for me, as the only tangible help for me—physical or emotional—would be the restoration of the normal functioning of my paralyzed extremities or, if that would never be possible, I would have to rely on my own inner strength and self-control.

This last illusion, however, was shattered at the moment of my academic retirement. In short, on that occasion I suffered what I had been observing in other, older colleagues for several decades; the sudden trauma of exclusion from the academic community that coincides with the bestowal of the title "emeritus professor." When it happened to me, I experienced what I had often observed in others with some incomprehension, the phenomenon of retirement depression. It once seemed so unreasonable to me, because, as I thought, these professors must have known from the beginning of their careers that they would have to retire and when the retirement would take place.

It is true, of course, that I too had known for years, months, and days when my academic career would come to an end. Nevertheless, like most of my colleagues, I shrugged off the awareness of my imminent retirement until the arrival of the very day when I also would be "honored" with the title "professor emeritus." On that day, the university gave a beautiful black-tie dinner in my honor with several affectionate speeches of good wishes, farewell, and appreciation of my scholarly achievements. I had been consulted about the guest list, and when I sat in the festive dining room of University House and looked around over my assembled friends, colleagues, and former students who spoke of me and to me with so much affection, I felt the familiar closing of my throat and moisture in my eyes.

I knew I was expected to get up and respond to the loving words of my colleagues; I also knew that I would not be able to do this with dry eyes, composure, and a steady voice. Throughout my life I have experienced leave-taking as an unbearable pain and tried to avoid it as much as I could. Even as a little girl, I changed the wording of a popular and sad children's song to give it a happy ending. The real text of the song dealt with a bird that came flying and perched on my foot to whom I was to sing: "Dear bird, fly on, take my greetings and a kiss, for I cannot fly with you, because I must stay here." As I never could bear to sing it with that finality, I had changed the words to reassure the bird and myself that I would be coming along after all.

Because, on the occasion of the dinner I still could not bring myself to say good-bye, I whispered to my husband, begging him to respond on my behalf to the various speakers of the evening. After he had done so with grace and gratitude for both of us, after the final applause of the evening had sounded, and the lovely party had ended, the guests filed past me one by one to shake my hand and to wish me well on my many future years of "leisure."

If there was anything I did not wish, nor do I wish it now, it is leisure. I wanted health and continued productive activity. As a consequence I have involved myself in many more projects than I can hope to complete before the respective deadlines arise on the calendar. This book, the completion of which is not tied to a specific deadline, is written from an inner need with the hope that by writing about my stroke and all the grief and pain it has caused me, I may be able to abreact some of my anger and resentment.

If this book were a novel or a fairy tale, I would have concluded it with the happy ending of a complete recovery; but since I have written a factual account, I must end it by admitting that I am still an invalid with unrelieved hemiplegia. At any rate, I came to expect that this condition would remain constant as the ultimate insult of my cerebral vascular accident. Instead, however, a new complication has arisen. Owing to the hemiplegia, and aggravated by my inability to engage in any physical exercise so that I have gained some weight in the last year, an increasing weakness of my left knee may have to be stabilized by a brace. The internist advises me to get fitted for a long brace now by the same orthopedic shop that sold me my first brace. By way of slim comfort, the physician told me that modern braces are much lighter and therefore more comfortable than those of two decades ago. Not happy at the need to return to a brace, I consulted the orthopedist whose successful operation of my shortened and contracted Achilles tendon freed me from the absolute need to wear my earlier brace. He remembered my previous dismay at having to cope with a brace and suggested that wearing one now is not an absolute necessity unless the present condition of my knee worsens.

Apart from this unexpected aggravation of my condition, I have been and am still leading a comfortable and rewarding life, largely thanks to my husband's serenity and equanimity which surrounds me day in and day out. My mood is marred only, since my retirement from my university duties, by a sensation of emotional and social isolation from my healthy friends and colleagues of former years. Most of them display great patience and helpfulness toward my impediments, but others find it difficult to deal with my recurrent melancholy. They suggest that with my successful career, my harmonious home life, and my beautiful home in the loveliest section of the San Francisco Bay area, I really have "nothing to complain about." In fact, I do not complain to anyone; it is only my emotional solitude that is sensed by others and is sometimes resented, since it is interpreted as a rejection and evokes a remoteness that leads to estrangement.

As long as I am concluding this brief epilogue with reflections on my emotional state, I feel I should add that I have freed myself of some of the awkward compulsion to weep at the slightest occasion. I am still quite ill at ease when I have to express sympathy to someone who has suffered a recent bereavement, because the disproportionate amount of my tears is apt to embarrass the mourner. For the same reason I also strictly avoid attending funerals or memorial services. When I see such services on television, such as a repeat showing of the funeral procession of President Kennedy in 1963, my grief turns to uncontrolled sobbing regardless of whether I am at home alone or whether others are with me watching the same sad event.

I have mentioned several times that although I may become accustomed to my permanent handicap I did not believe that I would become reconciled to it. Now that I seem to have gained some control over my emotional outbursts, I feel justified in hoping that I may also learn to control my frequent surges of irritability which constitute an ever-present threat to my social interaction with friends and colleagues.

While I have been deploring the loss of most of my skills and ambidextrous capabilities, I have been able to comfort myself over some skills that I had previously failed to acquire and therefore had not lost. Among those I think primarily of the nine years of my childhood and my adolescence during which I was to have become a violinist. As was customary at the time of my youth, my parents decided that I was to learn to play a musical instrument. I think I might have been willing and even eager to do so, had the instrument selected for me been the piano. But since my mother was a gifted musician and played the piano very well, it was decided that I was to play the violin so that she and I could enjoy playing duets together.

Somehow, I lacked the zeal and motivation to become a good violinist. My teacher's indifference to my musical progress made me dislike my own playing so much that I even avoided the practice sessions during which I would have had to listen to my own unmelodious playing. The few times my mother and I attempted to play a duet ended in mutual disharmony between us, because I was unable to maintain the correct rhythm in spite of the accompanying metronome.

It was almost a relief when at age seventeen and after nine years of futile violin lessons, I became severely ill of scarlet fever and was quarantined for six weeks, as was then customary. Afterwards I had to spend my time in making up for the schoolwork I had missed and the family decided I should stop playing the violin. The only vestige of those wasted years of tuition and minimal effort on my part are my love and admiration for good violin playing and an oil painting that shows me at age fourteen in a royal blue velvet dress, holding a beautiful, shiny, brown violin on my right arm and lap. Somehow, my parents had imagined that the existence of this portrait would awaken a spark of obligation in me to become the youthful artist who was so attractively pictured in that painting. But scarlet fever, an illness that has been mastered by the progress of medicine, had saved me from any desire to live up to the memory of the painting of the "Young Girl with Violin." During the Second World War, when our home, no longer inhabited by my family, was destroyed by a bomb, the oil painting and my mother's grand piano also vanished from this earth. Now that I have lost the use of one hand, I find it fortunate that I had not become a talented musician, for in that field the loss of one hand would have been devastating.

Another inverse boon of my handicap was that I had not followed my original professional intention of becoming a plastic surgeon, or for that matter, any kind of surgeon at all. The field of plastic surgery had attracted me even before I began to study medicine and, as a medical student, I spent every summer vacation as a *famula,* or personal apprentice, to a plastic and reconstructive surgeon. I was lucky inasmuch as I could draw quite well and design the surgical alterations that were to be undertaken. My pleasure in drawing and painting remained great when I succeeded in doing a number of fairly acceptable portraits of friends and family members.

Again it seemed I was fortunate that my plan of becoming a plastic surgeon was stranded on the fact of my gender, for there was no thought in the thirties that a woman could receive a residency or assistantship in surgery. So, my two youthful failures in life—artistry on the violin and the practice of plastic surgery—saved me from experiencing

Afterthoughts

two devastating results of my hemiplegia. It was fortunate that after coming to the United States I had chosen to become a medical historian, a field of endeavor I was able to carry on with one hand, and that I will be able to pursue as long as my right hand and my mind continue to function.

Glossary of Medical Terms

Achilles tendon. The powerful tendon at the back of the heel formed by the united tendons of the large muscles of the calf
Adrenal cortex. Part of adrenal gland that secretes hormones affecting growth and gonads
Aneurysm, aneurism. Dilation of a segment of a blood vessel, often involving the aorta or pulmonary artery
Agnosia. Loss of the ability to recognize sensory impressions, especially of touch, sight, and hearing
Angiogram. An x-ray photograph of blood vessels after an injection of a radiopaque substance
Aorta. Great artery arising from left ventricle, carrying blood from the heart to all parts of the body
Apoplexy. Stroke
Apraxia. Impairment of ability to execute movements to use objects correctly
Contracture. A permanent shortening of muscle, tendon, or ligament
CVA. Cerebral vascular accident
Disinhibition. Removal of inhibition or restraint
Electroencephalogram. The record produced by tracing of brain waves by means of electrodes placed on the scalp or in the brain itself

Facilitation. Lowering of the threshold for reflex conduction by the passage of a simultaneous stimulation from a reflex of a different origin

Foot drop. Also dropfoot. Contracted muscle of the calf

Gluteal muscle. Any muscle of the buttocks

Hemicrania. Headache on one side of the head

Hemiplegia. Paralysis of one side of the body

Hysteria. Neurosis involving symptoms characterized by lack of control over acts and emotions

Hemianopia. Defective vision or blindness in half of the visual field

Intravenous. Within a vein

Occlusion. Obstruction of the flow of blood

Physiatrist. Doctor who specializes in physical medicine, using physical agents in diagnosis and treatment (light, heat, water, electricity, etc.)

Proprioception. The reception of stimuli produced within the organism

Radioisotope. A radioactive isotope

Radiopaque. Opaque to x-rays or other forms of radiation

Scintillating scotoma. Blurring of vision with sensation of luminous appearance before the eyes, with zigzag, wall-like outlines

Spasticity. A muscle's continuous resistance to stretching due to abnormally increased tension. Suffering from spasm

Temporoparietal. One of a pair of broad, thin muscles of the scalp (also temporal parietal)

About the Author

Ilza Veith, M.D., Ph.D., studied medicine at the Universities of Geneva and Vienna. As a Rockefeller Fellow and with a grant-in-aid from the American Council of Learned Societies, she pursued postgraduate studies in history at Johns Hopkins University and received her doctorate in the history of medicine, the first such degree to be awarded in the United States. She taught in the University of Chicago's Department of Medicine from 1949 until 1963, when she was appointed Professor of the History of Medicine at the University of California, San Francisco Medical Center. Dr. Veith has served as Alfred P. Sloan Visiting Professor at the Menninger School of Psychiatry, Topeka, Kansas. Among her many books are *Medicine in Japan*, *Medizin in Tibet* (published in Germany), and *Hysteria: The History of a Disease*.